LOOK UNDER
THE SHEET

LOOK UNDER THE SHEET

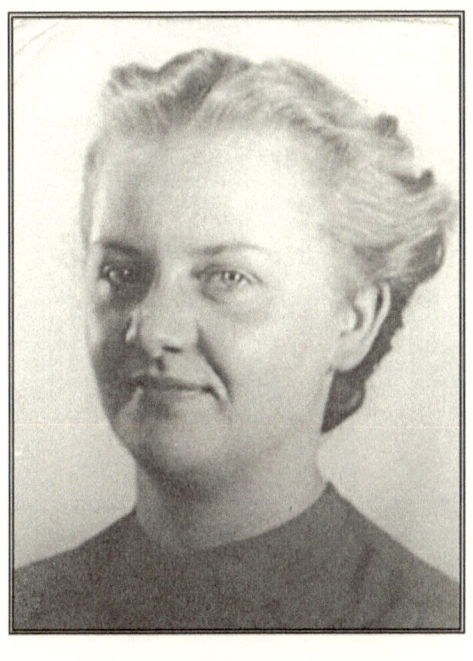

A Devotion to my Wife

GERARD van AMSTEL

iUniverse, Inc.
Bloomington

Look Under the Sheet
A Devotion to my Wife

iUniverse books may be ordered through booksellers or by contacting:

iUniverse
1663 Liberty Drive
Bloomington, IN 47403
www.iuniverse.com
1-800-Authors (1-800-288-4677)

ISBN: 978-1-4759-0284-6 (sc)
ISBN: 978-1-4759-0286-0 (hc)
ISBN: 978-1-4759-0285-3 (ebk)

Printed in the United States of America

iUniverse rev. date: 03/26/2012

CONTENTS

For Olof,

A good kid, a dedicated son, and an amazing, benevolent soul.

For Karen,

My strong-willed daughter with an enthusiastic
spirit and steadfast devotion.

Especially for Ellen,

My brilliant daughter whose remarkable
talents made this book a reality.

INTRODUCTION

My wife, Christina, first began having "problems" in her early fifties, which was around the year 1976. We were living in Wanaque, New Jersey where Christina was working at Prentice Hall while I was commuting to New York City. Christina began bringing her work home, because she was no longer able to complete it during her normal work hours. She became forgetful, and everyday tasks seemed to confuse her. At first I paid little attention and perhaps even attributed it to menopause or just the side-effects of the fifties. She never actually had a traffic accident; but, after a few instances of placing the car in drive as opposed to reverse . . . gas instead of brake, she eventually feared driving and had to resign from her job. At some time after her resignation, my company consolidated, and we sold our home and relocated to Louisville, Kentucky after an interim stay in a New York City apartment. The move to new and unfamiliar surroundings proved to be very stressful for Christina. The confusion increased exponentially. The doctor diagnosed Christina with dementia.

Even though the Alzheimer's Association was founded in 1979, I found it very difficult to find accurate information on this disease, especially information that related to such an early onset, and I found no information on what to expect or how I could best take care of my wife. I began writing as an outlet, as my salvation. I kept writing every day. I wrote about the daily stresses, the despair, and about moments of joy. I now want to share our story, our journey. If there are others seeking information as I was, I hope this book offers some answers, or more importantly some form of solace.

CHAPTER ONE

A Few Events in the Life of Christina van Amstel

"Our baby lies in her crib, looks up at the ceiling, and starts to laugh," I heard a young mother say. She looked at her baby and then at the ceiling. "Nothing is there, but the baby still laughs." She looked down at her baby. "I do not see anything, but maybe she does. Maybe she sees angels."

When Christina is in a blackout period, she lies in her lounge chair, her head tilted backward, with her eyes facing the ceiling and her lips open. Then suddenly she starts to laugh, sometimes really loudly. No one here, except for our children, ever knew Christina before she was afflicted with dementia. Even so, those who have met her know about her laughter. Even in the terminal stages of her illness, she will suddenly start to smile and then laugh. Could it be that Christina sees what we do not see?

What peace of mind; it is beyond our understanding.

One of our friends was planning a trip to the Netherlands. Christina asked her to visit Christina's mother. Once in Amsterdam, our friend found what she hoped was the right address and rang the doorbell. Christina's mother opened the door. Here were two women who had never met, standing face-to-face. Our friend explained who she was, and Christina's mother started to laugh. Our friend then knew she was at the right address. Their laughs are almost identical.

When Christina was in elementary school, she volunteered to take small children out for walks or push them in their baby strollers

1

through her neighborhood. Even as a youngster, Christina loved babies and taking care of children. Christina stayed in close contact with one of these children. On our first trip back to the Netherlands after emigrating to the United States, we visited this child, who was now a married woman with many stories from the blissful days when Christina took care of her. She lived with her husband in a beautiful old home on a dike that was wide enough for a two-lane road. This home is now protected as a historic landmark. On one side of the dike is land, and on the other side is a large lake, which used to be an inland sea. Small rowboats are moored there and move up and down as the waves roll in. Our friend took care of her mother for more than ten years, because no one else in the family would do it. She knows what it takes to care for an ill person.

Christina's love of babies continued into and throughout her adult years. It is no wonder that Christina became a private maternity nurse. Fifty years ago, in our home country, children were born at home. Expectant mothers went to their doctors but also hired a private maternity nurse. When the time came, they called the doctor; however, the nurse usually arrived first, so sometimes Christina delivered the baby.

I met Christina in the winter of 1944, during a meeting of young adults from our church. She was wearing her nurse's uniform. The southern part of the Netherlands had been liberated by Allied forces, but Amsterdam was still occupied by German troops. A few months earlier, an attempt had been made to capture a bridge over the Rhine River, but it had failed. That same winter, the Battle of the Bulge was fought and won.

The stores were closed and boarded up. There was no food, no heat, no electricity, no news. The only news came over radios controlled by the Germans; it told us that the Germans were still winning on all fronts. The only food the Germans allowed citizens to have was one loaf of bread a week. This bread was so bad that if you put the ends of the loaf between your hands and squeezed it, it became a wet gray ball. No one could survive on this food. Christina lived with her mother and her older sister. The sisters decided to go north to find a place to work for food; this way their mother would have three loaves of bread per week. They walked a total of eighty miles, stopping at the homes of relatives and friends along the way. With the help of pastors from local churches, each of them found a place to work for food. Their mother survived but had a severe case of malnutrition for quite some time.

After the war, Christina and I met again and started dating, but we were separated again by forces beyond our control. The unexpected surrender of Japan had created problems for the Allied Forces in the Pacific. There were not enough troops available to occupy the countries that Japan had captured during the war. The Netherlands had to supply troops to do their part in Indonesia. All males born in 1925 were the first draftees after the war. We were trained in record time and shipped to Indonesia. After a four-week voyage by ship, we arrived in Indonesia. One year passed, and then a second, a third, and then one more year. Christina waited all those four years and so did I.

During those years of separation, Christina found a very good job with an excellent salary, and each year she received a bonus of three months' salary. The company provided vacation homes at no cost to the employees. When I came back, we waited another year before getting married. Since she made more money that I did, she kept on working. In 1951, this was quite unusual. After four years of marriage, we had our first child, Olof.

Christina kept working as long as she could during her pregnancy. She enjoyed her regular visits to the doctor, as her manager arranged a company car and a chauffeur for each visit.

After Olof was born, we moved to America. Like most immigrants, we lived in rental homes, and as a result, we moved more than we would have liked. When a realtor who attended our church started a large new development across the highway, Christina said, "Let's buy a new house." My wife went to the builder as well as the realtor who financed this project, telling them our plans. The builder was an immigrant from Europe, and the real-estate office owners were members of our church.

My wife was raised in a family where owning a home was part of life. I was raised in Amsterdam, where most families lived in apartment buildings and the desire to own a home did not come into the picture. While in Minnesota, she found out what it would cost to have a home built, which included the mortgage payment and real-estate taxes plus a down payment. The mortgage payment on a new home was about the same as what we were paying to rent a home, but the catch was the down payment. My salary was just enough to cover the bills, with no money left for savings. We had to come up with a plan to get the money for a down payment. We canceled our health insurance for the whole family for one year to save the money. After a year of saving, we were still short by half. Christina worked out a deal with the realtor and the contractor. We would purchase the paint for the house and would paint it ourselves, inside and out, with one primer and two coats of paint. Christina was an excellent painter; I was the sloppy one. My wife painted during the afternoons, taking our youngest daughter, Ellen, along, while I painted on Saturdays.

We probably never would have had a home if we had not followed Christina's plan. When we built our new home in Minnesota, she let the contractor know that she did not like the traditional double-hung windows. Instead, she wanted casement windows for the living room. She wanted a large picture window, starting about fourteen inches from the floor, a hip roof, a full basement with a shower, and clapboard siding covered with soft yellow paint. We had oak trimming on all the windows and doors and oak flooring. It was an eye-catching home.

Shortly after we moved into our new home, Christina wanted to visit her mother. As it turned out, it was good that she did this, because about six months later her mother died in her sleep. It was difficult for Christina to travel, because she suffered from motion sickness and did not like to fly. We drove her to the local airport in our small town of Mankato, where she boarded a DC 3 to Minneapolis. From Minneapolis, she flew to La Guardia Airport in New York and then went by shuttle bus to Kennedy Airport. She left the United States in a four-engine propeller plane with a stop in Iceland. The total trip was more than twelve hours. I took care of our children, made breakfast, and got them ready for school.

After school they stayed with one of Christina's friends, where I picked them up and then made dinner. For four weeks I was a single parent, a term not yet in use.

When I graduated from Mankato State University, the son of the US vice president was in my class. His father was the commencement speaker. When Hubert H. Humphrey left after the graduation and was walking to the helicopter, Christina walked up to him and started a conversation. She told him that her husband was also graduating, and a conversation followed. As soon as others saw that Christina was talking to him, they overcame their shyness and came and shook hands and talked with the vice president.

At home after graduation, she surprised me with a college ring. We had talked about it but had decided not to buy one, because we did not have the money to spend. Later one of our children told me that "Ma" had sold one of her precious possessions and paid for the ring with the proceeds of the sale.

When we moved from the Midwest to the East Coast, Christina started to work again to help for the down payment for a larger home. Houses on the East Coast were three to four times more expensive than in the Midwest. We built another home with four bedrooms and three full baths in an excellent area in the New Jersey mountains.

Ever since we were married, we had both worked and shared the domestic duties. When Christina started to work again, we followed the same routine. I washed and ironed. In both summer and winter, I hung the sheets outside on the clothesline; in the winter, they froze solid in a minute. One day I could not find my college ring. We looked everywhere, but it was gone. A few months later, Christina was in the backyard when a shiny object caught her attention. She walked up to it, bent down, and picked it up—it was my college ring. I was very happy to have it back. It must have slipped off my finger when I had hung out the sheets that winter.

Years later, when Christina had to go into the nursing home, staff members and others would say, "We wish we could have more residents like Christina. If there were more people like Christina, the world would be a better place to live in." She was a flower and bloomed wherever she was planted or replanted, even though she did not like to be replanted. She was a person who gave spontaneously. It was a natural expression of her personality. It was her inborn beauty to make others happy. Her happiness let her laugh, even in the terminal stage of dementia. Her illness deprived her of many joys, but not her peace of mind.

CHAPTER TWO

Preparing for Retirement

Universal Declaration of Human Rights, Article 25

Everyone has the right to a standard of living adequate for the health and well-being of himself and of his family, including food, clothing, housing, and medical care, as well as necessary social services, and the right to security in the event of unemployment, sickness, disability, widowhood, old age, or other lack of livelihood in circumstances beyond his control.

Motherhood and childhood are entitled to special care and assistance. All children, whether born in or out of wedlock, shall enjoy the same social protection.

It was still years before our retirement, but we were already planning for it. We could not possibly stay in the same town—or the same state, for that matter—because real-estate taxes and our mortgage payment would take too much out of our pension check. Besides, this home, where we raised our three children, was too large for a retired couple.

We did not need anything fancy—central air-conditioning for the summer and a fireplace for the winter. We would also need a snow blower, since we had done enough snow shoveling, and a dependable car, one that would last us the remainder of our lives. Our friend had a Volvo and had put *one million miles* on it, so we decided that would be the make of car we would buy. We also planned to visit our relatives in the Netherlands and take a cruise to Curaçao.

The first thing we had to decide was which state we should retire in. We had lived in seven different states since we came to the United States, and we did not know where we wanted to end up. We did not like hot climates. We decided to travel to try to find our ideal spot. Since we had good friends in Minnesota and wanted to visit them and see the first home that we had owned, we started our travels with a trip back to Mankato.

When we drove down our old street in Minnesota, it looked so different. The trees and evergreens, which were small when we had planted them, were now large trees. Our evergreens had grown to about twenty feet high and were quite a beautiful sight. The new owners had changed the color of the house and installed an awning over the picture window. Then we went to the new airport. Only small private jets were parked, and just like the old airport, it was not busy. When we went to our old church, we discovered that our pastor had retired. We would not be returning to Minnesota.

The following year we took our Volvo on another road trip in search of our ideal retirement spot. We went to Maine, the Vacation State, and New Hampshire, and then cruised around the lower part of Maine. It was surprising to find the differences in that part of Maine and the vacation areas up north. Although the land was beautiful, it was a little rustic for our tastes and too remote from major highways. It was not a place for us to retire. Then we drove north and looked at different towns with accommodations to fit our purpose. The homes we liked we could not afford—the real-estate taxes were too high. So this was a nice, short visit.

In the fall of that year, we read the newspaper advertisements every Sunday about new developments in Pennsylvania. We selected a couple of builders and called them and made appointments to meet them. The developments were only half an hour's drive from each other. We received a letter with an invitation to come to their office and stay in a large hotel at their expense. We called back to set a date and time. First, the sales agent wanted us to see what was available immediately. It came close to the plan we had shown him, but there were always certain aspects of location, lot, and surroundings that we did not like. We told him that we wanted a curb and a gutter, since a nice neighborhood loses its attraction by not having a curb and a gutter. We also wanted sidewalks and underground power lines and did not want the lot to be too small. Recently developers had started providing larger homes, but those developments often looked crowded, with the large houses on small lots. To us, trees and landscaping provided value. The other requirement we had was public transportation to the nearest town.

When we drove into the development we were excited. It had wide streets, curbs and gutters, sidewalks, all electrical cables underground, an excellent street layout, and good landscaping. Some lots were level, but others sloped to drainage ditches, and the streetlights were great.

The development had been a small farm and was adjacent to the city limits. A real-estate company had bought the farm and made this the first large extension to the small city of New Holland, Pennsylvania. A two-lane highway ran through the town with bus services to the next larger town, the county seat. Right off the main road in this development was a section of condominiums in clusters of six units. Each had two bedrooms and a garage. Each cluster had different kinds of bricks. The landscaping was beautiful. The street layout used cul-de-sacs and slightly curved roads, and at the edges of the development, the homeowners could look from the backs of their houses to the surrounding farmland.

We went inside a couple of homes with one floor and also into a two-story home. You could see this was quality workmanship. We were impressed. But the homes in this development had small rooms and were built on small lots. When we mentioned this to the sales agent, he told us there would be one more section added after all the current homes were sold. These homes would have larger lots and more square footage. We told him we would be back when they started building on the larger lots.

Chapter Three

Unexpected Changes

For some time, rumors went around our office that our company might merge with another one. They had started as one company but had broken into two after the Civil War. They were not merging to heal old wounds; it was business, or more exactly, global business. The cost of office personnel was getting too high in New York City, where my company was located, and it would be better to find a cheaper labor force. Since the two companies were in the same business, quite a few people would lose their jobs.

The New York office was much smaller and did not have the latest equipment in administration and had a different management system. The other company, located in Richmond, was against the merger.

There was an announcement at a combined annual meeting, where the proposed merger was to be explained and then voted on. The result of that meeting was that the Richmond stockholders voted against the plan and it was defeated.

This was quite a relief, but how long would it last? People did not want to lose their jobs, leave friends and relatives behind, sell their homes, move children out of school, and uproot their whole world. For quite a while, there was no news. Then, a year later, another combined meeting was announced. By this time, almost everyone in the New York office had relaxed and did not expect any change, so it came as a great surprise when we heard that a merger had been approved by both sides. Preparations were already under way to have the merger completed within the next year. Who would be hired for the new company? Some said they wouldn't leave New

York City, while others would opt for early retirement. Quite a few employees indicated a willingness to join the new company if the conditions were the same or better, or to leave if the severance pay was generous.

The new CEO was appointed for a three-year term. He was from the Richmond company. The second-in-command was from New York with the same term. These appointments went into effect as soon as the legal documents were signed. The top two men selected their department heads, and these in turn selected the middle management, who had to fill all office positions. To fill all these vacancies as outlined in the transition policy, job postings were displayed on every bulletin board in the building.

I believe that a company has the moral and ethical responsibility to treat its workers according to written and verbal agreements, and use their skills and abilities so they can earn a standard of living to support their families.

In front of the bulletin board many opinions were expressed, especially when it came to the salaries of the managers. One of the main reasons for moving was the cost of labor; however, the salaries of the managers were not cut—they were increased. When it came to the office workers, it was just the reverse. These were the so-called "savings."

When I knew that I had a position in the new structure, our family had to make a decision. The sale of our home was the first priority. We had bought our home in 1970; twenty years later, the value of our home had skyrocketed. We called a local realtor, who came over and inspected our home and made an appointment to come back to quote a price and provide other information about the sale. After a week on the market, we did not get a response. I called our broker and told him to drop the price by ten thousand dollars. He said to wait, believing the set price was correct. But I knew we would have problems, and if it did not sell, the price must be the reason. Reluctantly, he agreed. Another ten days on the market and still no offers. I called him again, instructing him to drop the price another ten thousand. This time, he tried much harder to convince me that we would get our price, but we did not listen. Soon after this, we did get a call and a visit, and our home was sold.

Later it became clear why dropping our asking price was the right thing to do. The real-estate market had apparently reached the top and was leveling out. We had received seven times more than what we paid for the house, and dropping only twenty thousand dollars was the best move. Others in our office would not drop their price, listening to the "experts." It took them a lot longer to sell.

We had two small problems: our roof and radon. The buyers had requested a radon test and had a building inspector come in to look over the house. When the test was done, the reading was above the federal standard. The building inspector found a rafter in the attic that had a split. He talked to our lawyer about this, who told us that houses in New Jersey were sold "as is." After some talk, we agreed to have the radon test done for a second time, and the result was below the federal level. We did not pay for the repair, and the real-estate office, afraid of losing a good commission, offered to pay for the repair.

We could pay off our mortgage and buy our retirement home with the cash from the sale, buy a new car, and have some money left. Our family owed this all to my wife, who had had the foresight to buy our first home at the right time.

The location of our new headquarters was not yet decided. We heard that Louisville, which was revitalizing its downtown area, had made a direct proposal to the new board. A bankrupt company offered a concrete building and the land on which it was built for one dollar. The city would build a parking garage big enough to park not only the cars of all of our employees but also of employees of other companies that might build or rebuild in the area. The city would remove all nonessential partitions and walls in order to offer an open space for the office layouts.

The mayor and his development staff presented this proposal first to the new board and later to the employees of New York and Richmond. Such an offer was too good to turn down. It would save on the building costs and solve the parking problems. All the cost for this merger came from the reserves of the two companies.

The chairperson of the location committee resigned in protest. He wasn't one for progress, and the project seemed to proceed smoothly without him. Civil engineers examined the skeleton building and found it to be in excellent condition for an office building with elevators.

The staff who had accepted positions in the new company flew out to Louisville to meet with real-estate people, bank personnel, church leaders, and school representatives. We would also tour the city and see the building site, which showed just the skeleton structure. We left in the late afternoon from our office and took a bus to the airport for a short flight. We arrived late, and buses were waiting to drive us to a large hotel where we met our sponsors and had a light dinner. The remainder of the evening was filled with listening to information; after that, each couple was assigned to a local couple to talk and answer questions. We exchanged telephone numbers and were told, "Anytime you want to call us, do so."

The next morning, we toured the city. The downtown area looked completely revitalized. This was where our new office would be. We also visited a very large shopping center and spent some time looking at the stores. After lunch at the hotel, we went back to the airport to fly home.

Having accepted my new position with the company and selling our New Jersey home, the next decision for us was whether we should buy or rent. We really did not know what to do. My job was so hectic. We came to the conclusion that it would be better to rent first, and if we wanted to stay, we would take our time finding a new home.

The realtor in Louisville was eager to help us. We drove to new developments and went into models and some ready-builts for sale, but we knew what we wanted. We saw older homes, but these were too large for us. The newer ones had bedrooms in front of the house, and we did not like that. We asked the realtor if she had rentals available, and she drove us to a really attractive neighborhood. Only one side of the street had homes; the other side had a very large park with walks and many old trees. A hospital was only two blocks away, and the traffic did not come through this quiet street. The house had a porch, a small front yard and larger backyard. There was a kitchen, a fireplace in the living room, a full bath, air-conditioning, two bedrooms downstairs, and a large one upstairs. The owner lived next door and was willing to rent the house to us, since he had heard about our company's relocation to the community.

Our New Jersey home was sold, and the closing day was set. Moving for all employees in New York and Richmond was handled by a company that specialized in large transfers of households from merging companies.

There was a problem. We expected to go to Louisville right after the closing date, but I was told that I had to stay four weeks in New York to supervise the closing of our office. I told the new owners that we did not have a home anymore.

Our company owned several apartments on the Upper West side, close to the building. They were used to house overseas executives and their families when they visited the headquarters for business. We could park our car in a garage that used elevators to bring the car to different levels.

Christina did not want to live in New York City, even if it was just for four weeks. She was afraid of crime, especially muggers, and only left the apartment with me.

It was the only time in my career that I could walk to the office, and it took only ten minutes. I often walked home to prepare lunch. At dinnertime, we had an amazing choice of restaurants, all within a fifteen-minute walk from our building. When we came back from dinner, we would enjoy the courtyard of our apartment building. It was hard to believe we were in New York City.

This building complex consisted of a small city block. Two sides had ten-story apartment buildings, and the other two sides had a brick wall topped with a high cast-iron fence. The security was excellent. Wherever you walked, you could always see at least one security guard. It was very well lit at night, and cars could not drive into the courtyard. The landscaping was beautiful. Huge trees provided shaded areas, and there were plenty of benches to sit and talk with other friendly residents.

One day I came home from lunch and Christina seemed to be utterly confused. She did not know it was time for lunch. I did not know what to make of this.

The stay in New York was interrupted when we got a call from the movers asking us to come to Louisville to arrange our furniture in the rental home. We only had to indicate where the boxes and other furniture should be placed. So we flew down to Louisville, with all expenses paid by the new company. We stayed in a first-class hotel for one day, which my wife really enjoyed. At dinnertime, there was piano music in the lobby. The pianist was excellent, and after diner we stayed in the foyer and listened in comfortable chairs.

The trip to Louisville was a nice break for the two of us. Back in our New York apartment, the time seemed to stand still. My wife was different. I was under the impression that it was the shock of the transfer. After living for almost twenty years in our New Jersey home, she was close to retirement, deprived of the company of our children, and staying in a town she did not like. All these things were not easy for her to deal with.

The garage where we parked our car looked like an old warehouse with a large elevator that stored cars at different levels. On our last day in New York, our car was already parked out on the street. I signed a form and drove the car to a gate, which only could be used to load and unload small items. We put our suitcases in the trunk and other small items in the backseats.

We were happy to leave New York and took our time to enjoy the trip. We could travel it in one day, but we decided to stretch it to two days. We again stayed in the hotel that my wife liked so much with the grand piano in the foyer. The next morning, after our breakfast, we went to our rented house. Soon after we arrived, the crew came in a small truck and started to unpack the boxes and put the contents in the locations where we wanted them. At lunchtime, we paid for their lunches. In late afternoon, when all the boxes were empty, folded up, and put in the truck, we made our final inspection and expressed our appreciation to the crew. When they left, we went out to try the local diners. The chain restaurants here were quite different. After our meal, we went downtown to visit my new office building.

Louisville was an old city, but the revitalization was impressive. The sidewalks were very wide in order to allow plenty of room for all the shoppers. Brick planter boxes ornamented these walks at regular intervals; the flowers were bright and colorful, and the streetlamps were quaint eighteenth-century replicas.

The new corporate building park was located in the old warehouse district, close to the river. Years ago, barges laden with goods unloaded and stored their merchandise in these warehouses until it was ready to be shipped by rail. Most of the warehouses had been leveled; only the ones with sound structures were saved and used by developers for office building space. After our evening tour of downtown, we stopped for groceries.

We paid a visit to our landlord and his wife. They invited us to come in. We asked about public transportation, and he told us it was pretty good. There was a bus stop only five minutes away from our home, and it would take me to my office. The church was not too far, but you had to drive. It was a small building, and it looked like the churches you see in older books, except the walls were all brick. An addition had been built on one side of the church for the social hall, and the parking lot was next to that. The hall was larger than the church. Our first church service was that Sunday. When we had selected our seats, we looked around and noticed that quite a few of the worshippers were older. There were only a few families with young children. It was our experience that after the service, we followed the members to the exit door where the pastor shook hands and made a few short remarks but kept the outflowing stream of members going. We were always the first ones out and sat in pews close to the door. This would not happen that day because the pastor saw us coming in and invited us to the social hall to have coffee and meet some members of the church. We went to the hall, had coffee, and met the members of this church. Our first impression was good, and from that day we became regulars of the "coffee club."

CHAPTER FOUR

It Is a Different Story
When It Hits Home

Christina seemed to be more at ease in Louisville. The friendliness of our neighbors was comforting, but it was the church and its members who were the best medication. We have been members of many churches as we've moved from job to job and from state to state. This church had a large number of retired people, many of them doctors and surgeons. The younger generation was in the minority, but the two pastors treated everyone with professional and loving care.

Our company had a good health-care plan, which included a prevention program. It had a contract with a medical research institute, which conducted examinations that were quite different from regular physical examinations. Later, the contract was terminated and we could go to our own family doctor. The cost of these preventive examinations was fully reimbursed. We had yearly examinations, but this year, because of the reorganization and transfer, we missed them. In our new town we were not familiar with the medical system, so we asked some of the retired doctors at the church for their opinions. They suggested going to the medical center next to the local hospital.

The laboratory work was done first, and each of us was examined by a different doctor. As we were ready to leave, the doctor called me into his office and told me that my wife had dementia. Since I had never heard that word before and did not know what it meant, he explained to me that dementia is an umbrella word used to indicate a group of brain diseases that lead to the loss of mental and physical functions. There are two groups, disorders which can be reversed and the nonreversible group. It is also the most misdiagnosed and over diagnosed disorder of mental functions in older adults.

Most medical doctors did not know much about this disorder. Our own doctor in New Jersey had not detected it. I was under the impression that all of Christina's confusion was due to our transfer, leaving our home where we had raised our family, and preparing for retirement, along with the big shock of living in New York, which she did not like. In our new surroundings, she seemed to feel better, but she was different—and it was impossible for me to pinpoint what the difference was. We needed some new furniture, so we went shopping, her favorite pastime. Christina had excellent taste. On our recent trip to buy furniture, she was different. She did not express her opinion of the furniture she was buying and did not talk to the salesperson as she used to. We were not ready to accept the diagnosis and went on with our lives in our new town.

The town was expanding rapidly, and we were using the old beltway to get to the various shopping centers. We saw a large number of new developments as a result of this expansion. On our way back from a shopping trip, we went into a development and looked at the new homes. That was just the beginning, and looking at and walking into homes being built became a new pastime. There were so many sites that we called a realtor to help us find a home. Christina told me she wanted to retire here. I was happy about this, because to me this was a good sign. We made an appointment for a Saturday afternoon with a woman from the realtor's office. She took us to an impressive new development. The homes were beautiful and elegant. They had ornate entrances, sometimes with pillars, artistic framing of the main windows, not one roof line but several going in elegant angles and elevations. Lot sizes were average. The streets were constructed with curbs, gutters, and sidewalks, underground power lines, and no basements. The realtor called us whenever she had time for a Saturday appointment. This went on for quite a while. But my wife began to lose interest. I asked her if we should stop looking, and she agreed.

At Christmas time, our children came. We had found a hotel with a rooftop dining room that revolved slowly so that you could see the city and the river. Of course we had to show this to our kids and have dinner there.

We became part of the neighborhood. Neighbors on both sides of our house invited us to sit with them on their porches when we took our evening walks. They told us stories about the town and their families. One neighbor was an artist who was working in the summer to complete one or two hand-painted manger scenes. She explained, "It must stay a relaxing and fun activity." We went to her place quite frequently. Our landlord lived next door, and his wife would visit my wife during the day.

I had promised my wife that when we moved she would not have to cook anymore. Back in New Jersey, after shopping, we ate out. If our children were home at dinnertime, we brought home take-out meals, which satisfied them. On Sundays, we had Chinese food, not the kind you buy in the "to go" place, but made from scratch. I had become interested in Chinese cooking many years ago and bought a book, a wok with a heavy bottom, a ladle, a strainer, chopsticks, and all the necessary spices and condiments. I showed our family how to use them, and when we ate homemade Chinese food, only chopsticks were used.

It did not take me long to find out that cooking day in, day out, year after year must be a boring job. It takes a lot of time to prepare a meal and then cook it, and bring it to the table only to watch it disappear in a matter of minutes. I realized it was a frustrating and unrewarding part of a married woman's life.

Most evenings after dinner, we went to the porch and had our tea. We drank two cups with cookies or chocolates. In between, I did the dishes, using hot water and a brush and letting them dry. Back on the porch, it was so peaceful and quiet, with hardly any traffic. There were few pedestrians. The gentle sound of birds singing blended beautifully and melodiously with our peaceful and quiet time on the porch, but then suddenly all this would change. The roaring engine of a plane was approaching. We knew it would be a 747, not a passenger plane, but a very large parcel plane. It would pass to the left of us and always seemed very low. It passed over at about the same time each evening.

When it became silent again, the birds would resume their songs. It was at this time we would hear the mocking bird at the highest branch of a tree, imitating the other birds. My wife whistled very shortly and repeated it after some time, and then again and again, and waited and tried again. Before long, the bird seemed to respond to this sound; then she whistled again, and the bird picked it up again. It made her smile.

Across from our rental home was a very large, beautiful park with a spacious lawn and trees everywhere. Generally, only dog walkers were seen there, but sometimes we went across the street and followed the walking paths. There were no benches to sit down and rest, so we kept our walks short. It was so peaceful.

Christina liked to drink coffee, and I liked to watch planes take off and land. For this combined pleasure, we could go to the airport, which was close by. For new residents of the town, getting to the airport was confusing. I went the wrong way a few times until I found out that an unmarked left curve was the right way to get there. Parking was very easy. Since we were used to metropolitan airports, this was fun. It was a small airport; the terminal was only two stories high. The walk to the planes was a short distance, and the coffee shop was never busy. In fact there were hardly any people there except when a flight came or departed. After that, it became quiet all over the airport.

Work was hectic. To merge two accounting systems into one was not strange to me, as I had done it before, but the new manager was very demanding. We had a system where we could access the main computer and write our own programs. After the general ledger was run, the reports were printed, but ironing out the problems took a long time. I took the correction work home. My work was always on time. I did not like the new manager's personality. He was young, with no formal education, but he had the ability to do this job. It was unfair to my wife, in her condition, that the time I now spent at home was used to find mistakes made by others. One Saturday, I did not show up to work overtime, which in my opinion was not necessary. He called me at home and told me to come in. At that point in time, I made up my mind to resign. I had helped him to get the system rolling in a shorter time than planned and had done my best in this reorganization.

Shortly after I left, a former coworker called and told me that two persons were now doing the work I had done. It gave me a good feeling.

Now we were faced with the problems of where to retire and whether to buy or build a home. I asked my wife if she wanted to stay here, but she said she did not. I asked her, "First you liked it here, and now you want to leave?" She did not answer that question, so I let it go. We didn't have much time to look around anymore unless we found a home already built, but that was quite unlikely. Then I remembered that development in Pennsylvania that we had both liked. I called the real-estate broker and told him our situation and asked about the section with the bigger lots. He told us these lots were now available. He told us there were six lots left and we had to select from three model homes. He would mail us these plans. We set a date to meet him to select a lot and the model we liked. He made reservations for us in the nearby town. Now we had a start.

It was only five hundred miles. Most people would drive it in one day, but neither of us liked driving. My wife had told me some time before that she did not want to drive anymore. First, she told me that she did not want to work anymore, and I said, "That is fine with me; you don't have to work." She had started working to pay for our children's college, but that was now over. We could now live on my salary. Getting in the car, taking off, and letting the engine run was a good feeling. In those days, the speed limit was seventy-five miles an hour, and on this highway there were hardly any cars. We drove only about four hundred miles and stayed in a hotel. Then the next morning we left in plenty of time for our meeting to look for a lot and begin talking about construction.

We met Joe the realtor in his office and took his car to the building site. Suddenly the car stopped running. He tried to get it started again, but it did not work. He called his wife, using the home phone of a resident who lived nearby. It took some time;

but she came, and we drove in her car to the building site, where he introduced us to the woman who was in charge of the project, Angela. Joe went with his wife to make arrangements to get his car fixed, and Angela showed us the six lots that were still available. There were only two lots we liked for their location and elevation. The one that had the highest elevation was our first choice, but then we told her we wanted a full basement. She said that was not possible on this lot, because there were rocks that had to be blasted and that would be quite expensive. Right behind it was the second lot. It was on a street that looked out onto two farms. We selected this lot. We showed her the model we had selected to be built on this lot, and it fitted into their requirements, but we wanted to make some changes. First, we wanted to add two feet to the width of the garage and add a door in the back. The garage was only insulated on the side between the home and the garage wall. We added a fireplace and selected a method of heating and cooling called a heat pump. We wanted oak floors in every room except the kitchen, bathrooms, and hall, where we wanted tile. We wanted casement windows with low-energy glass. We selected a French door that opened to the patio, which we increased to two times the size shown on the plan. In the kitchen, we upgraded the cabinets to solid oak and made sure there was a cut-out space for our microwave in the cabinet area. We took some space off a large walk-in closet in the master bedroom and used it to install a shower, giving us two full baths upstairs. We added a full basement, which included a full bath and a radon system consisting of perforated pipes under the basement floor, with a suction fan to eliminate unclean air. We had ducts installed for air and heat to be used when the basement was finished. We worked to get this agreement done and ready to sign, but we still had to select the colors.

Usually my wife was the expert, but she said to me, "Why don't you do it?" These words reminded me suddenly and painfully about her illness. I asked Angela to help me select the colors, and she did a good job. It was time to sign the contract. Christina could not sign her name. I asked her, "Please try it." She did, but it was not her normal signature. We wanted to go back to the hotel, relax a little, and have dinner. There was, however, one important item to be discussed. We would not be present to watch the construction. I asked Angela to please give us a phone call when the framing was complete, and we would come and inspect it and make changes or adjustments.

It was late when we left her office. When we got back to our hotel we had dinner. After that we walked for some time, sat in the lobby, looked at the paper, and then went back to our room and relaxed.

The next morning we left early, because we wanted to travel most of our return trip on that day so that we would be home around noon on the following day.

On Sunday after the church service, we had our regular coffee hour with the churchgoers, talked about what we had done to get the construction started, and also told them that the person in charge of this large project was a woman. Some of them smiled and said this would be the first time that a contract would be delivered on time. I replied, "You have not met this woman" and left it at that.

We got our phone call telling us that the framing was done, and we told Angela that we would meet her at the site.

When we arrived at the building site, we had to find the best way for my wife to get into the house. We could not use the front entrance. The only way in was through the back door of the garage. Inside the home, we saw not the regular two-by-twos but six-by-sixes, meaning better insulation. The basement floor consisted of precast sections joined with bolts and insulation on the concrete. The basement floor was not poured, so we could see the perforated pipes of the radon system all over the basement floor and saw where they had come together to one solid pipe with an exhaust system to flush out the radon. The plumber was working in the bathroom, which included a shower, toilet, and vanity. Then we went outside to the backyard and looked at the exposed concrete wall of the basement. There was too much exposure at the end. We asked, "What will happen here?" This was the section under the French door. She told us that steps would be made only for the door. Our response was, "It will look very cheap." We proposed a change. Making a planter box as far as the edge of the patio and so wide that it would almost meet the edge of the French door and then constructing a platform extending three feet and as wide as the total length of the French door, with only one step going to the patio.

During the building of our first home, we had made movies of almost every step in the construction process, from the empty lot, to the hole in the lot for the basement, the basement walls, the wooden floors on top of the rafters, the walls, and later the inside. This time we took only pictures of the walls, especially the six-by-six studs, and some interior pictures.

During the construction of our retirement home in Pennsylvania, we had some small problems resolved by telephone conversations.

Chapter Five

Retirement Not as Planned

For the first time in my professional life, we had to pay for our moving expenses. We made calls to various movers. Quite a few did not even call back, but we did get one who came out, looked at our furniture and closets, and prepared an estimate, with details about packing, loading, and transfer time from our current location to the new one. He told us there would be more than one household in the van.

We had to arrange for the closing of our new home in such a way as to be ahead of the movers. We had a yard sale and sold what we really did not need in the new home. What we did not sell we gave away by putting a sign up that said "Free," and it all disappeared.

Moving day arrived. The movers were here to pack our belongings, maybe for the last time. Moving and packing days were always messy and confusing, leaving you lost in your own home. The next day they loaded all we had in the van; it was not really that much. It was late afternoon when they closed the doors on the van.

Our neighbors came to say good-bye. We took pictures of them with my wife. We drove out of Richmond onto the highway on our way to our new home.

We took our time on this trip. If we saw a large shopping center, we stopped and spent time there. We also called our real-estate broker and told him that we on our way to the hotel where we stayed every time we came to town, and he told us he could get us a company discount.

The day before the closing, we had our walk through. We tested the water pressure by letting one faucet run and watch that flow and then turning on another one in another part of the house to see if the flow in the first one stayed the same. We turned on some lights, tried some of the appliances, and flushed toilets. We had a one-year warranty with the construction company for any issues. The lawn looked terrible. It was hydro seeding and looked like a papier-mâché carpet, with black hoses running from the downspouts to the sidewalk. There were two trees, one in the front yard and another in the backyard. But we knew it was only a matter of time before the lawn took hold and the trees grew.

The next morning we had the closing at our lawyer's office. The documents were signed and checks were presented to make this purchase legal. My wife had problems with her signature but we took our time. This only reminded me again about her illness. We got the keys to our home. We left the office and went straight to our house. We unpacked the camping equipment we had brought along so we could sit or lie down. We had also brought some pots and cups.

We finally made it! Retired, after many years of working and saving. However, there was a dark cloud hanging over all this. Neither of us had ever been ill. Now Christina had this unknown illness about which we knew nothing. What I knew for sure was that my wife was different; she spoke very little. She was not who she used to be. This was a very unhappy experience at a time of our life that should have been happy for us. Our children were finally all on their own, a privilege that came very late for us. We had never had the empty-nest experience. Now we had the home we wanted and were happy to finally have a home of our own again.

The next day the movers would arrive to unload. The unpacking would be done by a local crew and our son would be there to help us. In past moves, Christina had overseen everything, because she always knew the best and most tasteful arrangements. All our children seem to have inherited this gene from their mother.

After all the large pieces of furniture were in place, the boxes were put in the rooms where they should be unpacked.

Before we moved in, I had walked down the steps to the basement and looked at the grain of the pine and said to the contractor, "Do not put any paint on these steps. I will put clear varnish on them." This was the first thing I did before we marked up the steps. I varnished first one side of the steps, and then the other side. The final project was to finish half of the basement for our children when they came to visit. The last job could only be done after I had had surgery on my hand. Since I knew this would be the case, we had taken a year of full medical benefits from my company after I retired. After my hand surgery I finished half of the basement. It was excellent therapy for my right hand and right finger.

It was a challenging job. There was an I-beam running lengthwise which had to be covered with wood so it could be used as a three-by-four. The carpenters who built the house had put two-by-sixes on top of the I-beam and driven nails at regular intervals; then they hit each nail on the side until it bend over the top of the I-beam, keeping the wood in place. I could not do this because the sides had to be level, so I drilled holes through the I-beam and wood.

I took many coffee breaks to see how Christina was doing. Sometime I brought her down to the basement. There was a chair on which she could sit and watch me work. If she went upstairs I quickly walked behind her and closed the door to the basement. She never came down on her own.

Ducts for heating and cooling were installed, so I had to make an outlet in the ceiling and connect that to the existing duct.

Every day we went out for a walk in the morning, in the afternoon, and in the evening. Each walk was about forty-five minutes to an hour. After daylight savings time ended, we eliminated the evening walk. We always walked hand-in-hand.

Long before we had retired, we were visiting one of those restored towns in a state park. We had walked a very long distance and wanted to rest. We found a bench where one other person was also resting. After a time, he started a conversation and asked, "How long have you been married?" I answered, "It will be forty years." He did not answer quickly but then he said, "You must love each other a lot." Then he walked away.

When it was raining, we dressed for it and took our umbrella along. If it snowed lightly, we put our snow boots on. At that time I had to dress Christina before going out.

You could get onto the patio from the back door of the garage or through the French doors from the dining room. The builder had originally wanted to make two steps to go down to the patio. I told him we were getting older so that might not be such a good idea. We told him to make a platform extending at least three feet out at the same level as the dining room floor with rails on both sides; it looked much better than the builder's idea. In the afternoon we used the patio umbrella to shield us from the sun and we had our tea there after our walk.

Christina liked to go to shopping centers. We had been so spoiled in the metropolitan area; it was a culture shock to come to a rural area where there was only one mall in the nearby city. It was small compared to what we were used to.

Our old shopping routine had been that each one of us went to the stores we were interested in. Now it was better that we stayed together. Christina might get lost, and trying to find her or calling her over the P.A. system would not do any good. There were plenty of rest areas to sit down and watch the shoppers go by.

There was a need in our area for persons to help out and prepare meals for the elderly and others who were not able to cook anymore. I called and joined the Meals on Wheels organization. I asked if it Christina could come and help, too. The task was to prepare sandwiches and fill plastic containers with food, but it had to be ready at a certain time so the drivers could pick it up and deliver it in time to the recipients. I found out that she was not able to do this. I should have known, but it takes a long time for an illness like dementia sink in. I had to get up early in the morning and leave her alone in the house. I was not comfortable with leaving Christina alone, so I stopped volunteering for the meals program.

We also joined two senior citizens groups. Their meetings were always at noontime once a week and started with a lunch, which was prepared by the members.

Once a month our small group went to eat in different restaurants in the area. This way we found out a lot more about this small rural area and also learned how to find our way through the country.

One time when we were eating with the restaurant group, I noticed that Christina did not touch her meat, but she ate all the other food on her plate. I observed this and got the idea that she was probably afraid to cut the meat, so I did it for her. I cut it in little pieces that she could handle, and she ate most of it. This is another one of those little things that mark dementia patients. Little by little they do not remember how to do things they have done all their lives. For example, Christina used to help me fold the bed sheets in the basement where we had plenty of room; one day she could not do it anymore.

At our senior citizen group meeting, there was usually a speaker after the meal. They spoke on various issues related to our interests. This was very boring to Christina, who could no longer understand the words of the speakers. The state she was in was just like a baby when it is born; its eyes are fully developed but it does not recognize the person it sees as its mother. After a short while we stopped going to the senior meetings. We went to other places that were not far from our home. There was plenty to see that was in close proximity to our home. We also found more shopping centers, and we walked in the malls in addition to our daily walks. Our doctor confirmed that exercise was important. We were always on the move, but we also took coffee breaks in the malls.

Every week a local newspaper wrapped in a plastic bag landed on our driveway. I always checked it for special events. One week there was an article saying that the local high school would have a "Colonial Day." Instead of taking our morning walk, we drove to the high school and parked our car. We went inside first but the pictures and posters of this event did not interest Christina, so we left the building and went outside. The first thing we saw, which could not be missed, was a very large black pot, suspended with a chain from a tripod. A fire was burning under the pot. So we took a closer look and asked, "What is this? What are you making?" We were told that this was how apple butter was made. A large wooden spoon was used to stir the pot, and it did smell good. We had heard of apple butter but had never tried it. It was delicious and we added it to our breakfast spreads.

The next stop was a place where a woman was spinning wool. I had heard about this art, which requires great skill and sensitivity of the fingers to get a perfect thickness. We watched the spinner for quite a while; she did a great job. The finished product on the spool was regular in size all the way around. When she needed to get a new supply of wool, she stopped, and while she was teasing the raw sheep wool to get it in shape for spinning, I asked her, "Do you sell the wool or do you use it for your family?" She replied, "I knit sweaters but I do not have any samples here. I am wearing one I made. If you are interested, I have patterns at home from which you can select." She gave us directions how to get to her home way out in the country. My wife's eyes were smiling at the spinner, which made me feel happy.

A couple of days later we went to the woman's home. It was off the beaten path in a lightly wooded area that was sunny and inviting. There was a little girl playing on the porch, and she was too busy with her play to be disturbed. We knocked and entered. We went through the living room into the dining area and out to the yard. Behind it was a meadow where we saw the sheep, the producer of the material for my wife's sweater.

We went back inside and the spinner took out a magazine with many sweater designs. Christina and the spinner selected a pattern and the proper buttons for this sweater. We asked, "How much will this cost?" She said, "Spinning the wool, preparing it for use and time for knitting will be one hundred dollars." We agreed on that and were told she would call us when it was ready. Then she took the measurements. I asked her to make the sweater roomy.

When we got her call, I asked if it was convenient for us to come in the morning around eleven o'clock. When we entered her home, she showed us the sweater; it was fantastic. My wife put it on and it fit perfectly. I asked, "Can you also make one for me?" I liked it that much. "I want a zipper instead of buttons."

She had talked to a friend about this sweater project and she told us that a hundred dollars was not enough money if you counted the hours of spinning and knitting. She made the minimum wage, and that was not right. She said she would have to raise the price to two hundred. I did not mind. *Two sweaters for three hundred dollars, all handmade from the start, was still a good price for this quality of work; they would outlast us.*

The second sweater did not take as long as the first one. We used the sweaters that winter. They were so heavy and warm. If you took the sweater off for a short while and put it back on, it was still warm. You do not have that with machine-made sweaters. These handmade sweaters were fantastic.

We walked every day, rain or shine or light snow. We always took the same route so as not to confuse Christina. The people in the neighborhood saw us three times a day, month in, month out; year in, year out. We walked together, hand in hand, or later, arm in arm. We had to cross streets and had to step off the curb to the pavement. One day I noticed that Christina was hesitant to step off the curb. We stopped and she looked down at the pavement, but she would not move. I did not know what to do, so I held her hand and stepped down while she remained on the walk. I encouraged her to come to me; finally she did, but the way she did it was strange. I got the feeling watching her motions that she was very scared. We took our time and when the she finally made the step off the walk onto the pavement; I got the idea that she had lost depth perception. She must have felt as if she was stepping into a hole. When this happened the second time I realized that this was another step down, literally and figuratively, in her illness. From that point on, in we stopped using the curbs. I looked for driveways which did not have an edge but a low decline to the pavement.

One morning as we were getting ready for our walk, I left Christina in the front foyer because I had left my keys in our room. It was a short distance, only fourteen steps, to the bedroom. I found the keys and went back. When I got to the hall she was gone.

Coming to the front door, I saw Christina lying on the short walk to the driveway. I did not hear the storm door slam, and she had made no cry for help when she fell. She was just lying there in an uncomfortable position. I bent down. She had her eyes closed and did not respond. I went back into the house and took a pillow from our bed and put it under her head and called 911. It did not take long for the ambulance to get there, because it was a small town. Christina was placed on a litter, her body strapped and her head secured, and we went in the ambulance to the hospital. While we were driving, she vomited. She could not move her head or bend over, which most people do when the vomit. So I asked, "Can't you put her head over to one side so she does not choke on her own vomit?" No response. I was angry. In the emergency room, she vomited again just a little. The nurse cleaned her up. She was taken to X-ray. I requested to be with her and explained that she had very advanced dementia and could not speak or react to instructions. I was allowed to watch in the observation room while she was X-rayed.

I was not only angry but also upset to find out that the hospital staff was not trained to handle patients with dementia. In those days, some had heard about Alzheimer's disease, but in the medical world, it was still the new kid on the block. Some doctors in the sixties, seventies, and even in the early eighties still used the term "hardening of the arteries." If doctors in those days did not know about this illness, how could you expect the other hospital staff members to know about it?

After the X-rays and examination, the doctor told me that she had a slight concussion. Rest was needed. I called one of our friends, who picked us up from the hospital and drove us home.

After this incident we never used the front door anymore. Nobody knew if it had been her lack of depth perception or if she just blacked out. I went to the lumber yard and bought a thick piece of plywood. I made a ramp to the garage from the side door so Christina would not have to go down steps.

We could not eat out anymore, so it was my turn to cook. The microwave pressure cooker was my favorite cooking pot. It had been a gift from our daughter one Christmas. It replaced the old-fashioned pressure cooker made of heavy metal that I had used when were just married because I was home first and had time to prepare a meal. I was very happy with this gift. In the box was a small booklet with recipes. Adding a small mixer to the pressure cooker gave me all I needed.

Now I had to feed Christina. I put the food on a spoon, brought it to her lips, and pushed it in slowly until she accepted it. She ate heartily. I gave her beverages through a straw. It was a time-consuming job. I fed her first and then fed myself, which did not take long.

Like so many women of her age, she preferred the tub to the shower. So far she had managed to take baths on her own; I filled the tub and she took it from there. On day I came to drain the tub and the water was just as clear as when I had filled it. She did not say anything. Her speech was already very limited. The next day, I helped her to sit down in the tub by telling her what to do. "Step with your right foot into the tub, then your left one, and hold on to the shiny bar on your right. Then hold the outer edge of the tub and sit down. Move down slowly and stretch your legs." I washed her and dried her and helped her to dress. There was not any problem. I dressed her sitting down on the edge of our bed. I helped her with her bra and top first, and then her panties in which she had a liner. Then we put on her stockings and her slacks and shoes. It was warm in the bathroom, but she was always cold, so I brought a small electrical heater with a fan and warmed up the bathroom. It was over eighty degrees. I perspired, but she was still cold. There was not much more I could do. I changed the routine after drying her off. I put the towel on her, let her sit down on the toilet, lid down, and dressed her there. Then she walked around the house.

She walked from the bedroom to the kitchen, into the dining room, into the living room, through the hall, and back to the kitchen. She kept this routine going. She did not walk slowly, but at a good pace. This went on and on. I had to get used to it. Our doctor had told me to let her walk. If I had had to explain to her what to do, she would not have understood it, but she managed all by herself. This exercise in the house was in addition to our regular three-times-a-day walk in our neighborhood.

We discovered Longwood Gardens and liked it so much we bought a membership to the park. It was a delight to see all the beautiful colored flowers. There was one small fountain with a few benches on which we always sat down to rest and enjoy the plants and flowers. There was also a small pond, and around it the flowers of the seasons. We walked up the steps to the exhibition hall, which most of the time had water in the lowest level and all kinds of palms arranged in a very artistic way. From the exhibition hall you could see the gardens with their breathtaking flowers in all kinds of colors and arrangements. We walked the Cascade Pass, a passage with tropical smells, moist and warm, and banana trees, and then we walked back to the gardens.

In the spring and fall we walked around the outside displays. We visited the Peirce du Pont house. The first name of the house was attributed to the Quaker farmer who had purchased the small brick house and sold it to the du Ponts, who extended the home for family and guests. The two magnolia trees in front of the house were quite an attraction because of their beauty.

After the visit to the house we would walk to the Italian water garden. The layout of this garden was inspired by a visit Mr. du Pont took to Italy. He was inspired by Italian gardens he'd seen, but he designed the water system to his own liking. The changes made in later years were corrected and restored to his design of 1956. It recirculates 4,500 gallons of water each minute, through six hundred jets of water, and is now computer operated. We spent plenty of time watching this beautiful display of water. It seemed to have a song of its own, like the movements of a ballet group. From the Italian water garden we walked the shoreline along the large lake that entered the flower garden. It required going down steps. I watched Christina's steps and held her close to me. From there, we walked back to the visitors' center and went to the restrooms before our ride home.

In the beginning of the year there were recitals in the ballroom at Longwood Gardens on an organ with ten thousand pipes. All the pipes were hidden behind a wall on the right side. Sometimes you could see the fabric move. This was caused by the volume of the air going through the pipes. I enjoyed the music, but I never cared for it when the organist did a lot of talking before each piece.

On some days, after our dinner, we went for a ride, traveling the country roads around our town. The highway had only two lanes and was not designed to carry the load of traffic it now had. Years ago plans were made to accommodate the traffic by building a new highway in a different location. It started by building a highway with two lanes in each direction from the nearest town to farmland outside the town. Some farmers sold, but others changed their minds after political pressure became so strong to preserve the farmland and the project came to a stop. However, time does not stand still. Small farmers made good money by selling their property to developers, and the influx of newcomers to this area had increased. It was a good place to raise a family, away from the large city. Schools were good and the area maintained a touch of rural life with the convenience of large-town shopping and entertainment.

My wife's favorite soap opera was *As the World Turns*. She had lost the ability to turn on the television or find the correct channel. In the past, she had told me about some of the players, but I had not understood how anyone could get addicted to a television show. But now, it did not take long for me to find the show entertaining, and time seemed to fly. Before I knew it, I was also addicted and we rarely missed a show. During the commercials, I made tea.

After the show we went for our afternoon walk. We frequently took a break in a memorial park. There were no fences, the trees had just been planted, and some work still had to be done to finish the detailed landscaping. Just before we had moved into our new home here, the spot was used by residents to plant vegetables or grow whatever they wanted to grow. We would sit on a bench where we could see the remainder of the park. The cows were in the field.

We took plenty of time to rest, and then we would walk home, hand-in-hand.

After our evening meal or ride in the country, our evening entertainment was *Wheel of Fortune,* then *Jeopardy* and the local news.

CHAPTER SIX

Seeking out Help

I heard about a support group for Alzheimer's caregivers. My son and I wanted to go but we did not have anyone to stay with my wife. Our pastor found a solution for this. He talked to the women's group from the church and they agreed to send one of their members to our house to watch my wife each time we went to a meeting.

We got a call from one of the members of the Women's Association. Since the meeting started at seven o'clock on Thursday evenings, I asked her to come over so I could explain a few things about how to assist Christina. I did not know how my wife would react to seeing a strange person in her home. When the lady came it was a relief to see that she had a very nice and easygoing personality. Christina seemed fine and I was happy to see the woman. I told her that there was a music tape ready to play, and there were a few more, if she needed them.

The support group met once a month at 7 p.m. It took me a little more than half an hour to drive to the nursing-home complex. At the time I attended these meetings, Alzheimer's was still an unknown illness to most of the population. There was not much help available to this group; it came much later. The caregivers were people in great need of help.

Most other illnesses were well known to us and we knew how to deal with them, but Alzheimer's was strange and disconcerting. Everything was new to us. We never felt at ease. We only repeated what everyone else told us about this disease. There are no pills, no surgery or radiation that can cure Alzheimer's disease. The research money spent on Alzheimer's disease is shamefully low. Other illnesses get much more attention. Alzheimer's patients cannot demonstrate in front of the White House or be very active in petitioning for more money. It is a silent minority that suffers needlessly. Few fight for the rights of the nursing-home patient. The nursing homes have turned this illness into a large money maker. Invest your money in this industry and you will be well rewarded by the return on your investment. A nation is not judged by how well it treats the rich but how it takes care of its poor, ill, and needy, young and old. Our nation would get a failing grade.

Dementia is an umbrella word used for the many, many brain diseases. But the only one known by the public is "Alzheimer's disease." Alzheimer's is the third largest killer. It is more feared than heart attacks and cancer. For the first two big killers, early detection can make the difference. Ninety-five percent of early cancer detection can save lives. If you have Alzheimer's, it is fatal. It is terminal.

For Alzheimer's, a preliminary diagnosis can be made. It involves a thorough mental and physical examination. It should include:

1. A thorough patient history
2. A complete physical examination
3. A psychiatric interview
4. The patient's medical history
5. A neurological examination
6. An exhaustive series of laboratory tests and diagnostic studies
7. A careful dietary analysis
8. A review of the patient's daily activities

All these tests have to be completed because there are diseases that mimic Alzheimer's. There is no specific test or finding that is unique to Alzheimer's. This process is called diagnosis by exclusion. Alzheimer's disease is: *not* a natural part of aging, *not* easily diagnosed, *not* limited to the elderly, *not* currently curable, and *not* covered by government, state, or federal funding.

There are many theories about this illness, including:

1. Chemical theories
2. Genetic theories
3. The autoimmune theory
4. The slow virus theory
5. The blood vessel theory

The only way Alzheimer's can be conclusively determined is after death by an autopsy of the brain.

At support group meetings, you can not only find a lot of information about this illness, but also get support from others who have similar problems. You are *not* alone. You have company and caring friends.

The Kassebaum/Kennedy law is a typical example of how unfairly we the citizens of this country are treated. Besides cutting down on reimbursements for medical treatments, this law also forbids the legal profession to advise us, the citizens of this country to use the existing laws to protect our assets from the results of catastrophic illnesses, which we cannot control.

Our human rights are violated according to article number 25 of the Human Rights bill which the United States of America has ratified. Congress pretends they are the defenders of freedom.

I found the sharing time at the meetings to be the best part, especially when the group members had the same basic problems in taking care of a loved one. One thing was clear: it is more difficult to take care of an adult man who has reverted to baby-like behavior than an adult woman. When the women talked about their husbands after they were diagnosed with Alzheimer's disease, I soon realized what a difference it was to take care of my wife.

Each support group meeting started with reminders and announcements. One evening there was a new item, "respite." We were told that we as caregivers could get respite twice a month for four hours at a time to be paid for by the support group. After the meeting I asked what I had to do to get this respite. It was simple. As I was a regular member, the group would submit my name to the organization that provided this kind of service for caregivers in general. First, I got a phone call from this organization and later I got a call from the nursing aide who would come to our home to take care of my wife from 1:00 p.m. to 5:00 p.m. It was an extension of the respite I already enjoyed from our church women, who cared for her while I was attending the support group meeting.

When the nursing aide came for the first time and met my wife, there was a great rapport. They liked each other. I told my wife that I would go and do some shopping and be home around five. Now it was my turn; I had to go out shopping for the first time without her and spend four hours. Nearby shopping did not offer much, so I decided to go to the next larger town, about a forty-five minute drive. Most of the time when we went to this shopping center together, the highway did not have a high volume of traffic. No one seemed to pay any attention to the speed limit. There was plenty of room, no crowded lanes. In the shopping center, my first stop was the coffee shop where I had a cappuccino. After that, I went to the tool and hardware sections of the larger retails stores. I did not feel at ease because the experience was so different. I went to a couple of other stores but found I had no interest, so I decided to go home. I did not drive fast. When I came to our own town, I stopped at the grocery store and bought a few items.

At home everything was normal. My wife was walking around the house in her usual pattern. I was told by the nursing aide that there were no problems. We talked for a short time and then I signed the paper that verified that she had done her job and said I would see her again in two weeks.

In Holland, there are two official Christmas days. Services are held on both days, but we did not have to go to church on the second. When I was a boy, we had a Christmas tree that was purchased on Christmas Eve and decorated at night by our parents with real wax candles. At night, after dinner, the lights were dimmed and each wax candle was lit. They were placed in such a way that no other branch of the tree could catch fire. It was a beautiful sight as we watched them burn slowly. The candles were not straight but had a spiraled outside surface, and as they burned, the wax started to drip first on the candle holder and then on the branch. I always watched in awe until the candle burned down so low that it had to be extinguished.

It was a great sight to see all the wax drippings on the branches and sometimes on the branches below them. No presents were given or received. We did sing some Christmas songs after this event, and then we would take from the branches chocolates rings or rings made from sugar with sweet liquid in them. Special meals were prepared on both days, usually rabbit or chicken.

When Christina and I wrote our parents about the Christmas customs here in America, we received parcels. Our children were excited when the mailman delivered the box. They knew that their grandparents always sent great gifts. They had seen their grandparents only in pictures. In one of these parcels, we got some vinyl records with music from our home country, songs for our children and organ and classical music for us. My wife and I loved listening to music. We both played the piano and organ. But Christina especially loved the music, and it had the power to soothe her.

Sometimes Christina would leave the room we were sitting in. It would take some time before she returned. She did not use the bathroom so I wanted to find out what she did. One evening when she left the living room, I followed her in such a way that she could not see me except if she turned around. From the living room she went into the foyer and turned into the hallway, which went to the bedrooms. She entered our bedroom and I waited. I looked in the room and she slowed down, walking very slowly. She passed the walk-in closet, but she continued very carefully and stopped exactly at the opening to the bathroom. Then she slowly moved her head little by little past the door jamb until she could look into the bathroom. Her body was not in the bathroom yet. It took quite a while before she actually stepped into the bathroom, and then I left. I went back to the living room and sat down. She returned through the kitchen to the living room and drank what was left of her tea. Then I went to the bathroom and found a cookie on top of the vanity. Sometime later, I found a chocolate and one more time

41

another cookie. She also brought her empty tea cup and put it on top of the vanity.

One day when she was in another room I did exactly what she had done, leaning against the wall and moving my head slowly. Of course, I saw my head in the mirror, but what did she see in her advanced stage of illness? She did not see herself, but a person she was not able to recognize as herself. Her brain had stopped this process of recognition. What we all take for granted did not work for her anymore. It did not scare her. She saw a person she liked. She did not know her and wanted to give her a cookie.

No one will ever know what went on in her mind, but one thing is for sure: It was an act of kindness. Caring for another person and giving away what she had at that moment was a token of friendship. This is what she was before her illness and what she still is in her illness.

Once, when we were in the kitchen; she was standing with her back to the refrigerator door and slowly went down to her knees, sliding down the door. She did not fall, but was sitting on the floor. I bent down and said, "Get up slowly," and supported her in her effort. It took some time and I had to repeat a few times, "Get up," and together we did it. The kitchen chair was only a few feet away. She rested on that chair. I made coffee. We each drank a cup. After that, she walked away.

On another occasion, I found her in the living room on the floor, sitting between her recliner and the oak chest, which was one of her favorite pieces of furniture. She must have felt one armrest and sat down. This time I could not get her up and said to her, "I will be back. I am going to get our neighbor Ralph to help get you up." He was at home. I told him what had happen. He came over. We lifted her up and put her in her recliner, where she had intended to sit. I thanked him, but she wanted to get up. We helped her and she walked away. It happened only two more times, and every time our neighbor was at home to help me get her up. Strangely, after these events, it did not happen again. She never made any sound when this occurred. Her speech was very limited.

One morning, I had her bath ready. She stepped over the bathtub edge, but did not sit down. I said, "Now you have to sit down," but she did not. I tried a couple more times and then it hit me. She had forgotten how to sit down. We all accept this routine as normal, but her brain did not give her the instructions anymore. Later, I tried getting in the tub myself and sitting down in it. We do it without thinking. It goes automatically, but to write it down is different. There must be more than one way to do this. So from that morning on, I washed her standing in the tub. Soon after that, she had problems getting her feet over the edge. I helped her, getting one leg in the tub while she was holding onto the safety bar and then getting the other leg in. It was really scary. I knew this was the first and last time I would do this. The tub had an anti-slip bottom, but still it was too risky. After this, I washed her outside the tub, sponged her top off, and dried her. She was one of the lucky ladies who did not have body odor. I put a towel over her and washed the remainder. I dried her off in two stages. First I dried the lower part of her body, and then I put her on the toilet seat and dried off her legs and toes.

Since my wife's illness, we had extra night lights in our bedroom. One night I woke up and turned to the right and she was not in bed but lying on the floor. She did not make any sound and probably was still sleeping. I talked to her and helped her up and checked to see if there were any signs of cuts or bruises, but I could not find any on her face or arms. She slept as usual for the remainder of the night.

The next day we went to a large department store to the children's section to buy a small bed rail with moveable rods to be put under the mattress. We could not find them and talked to the manager and explained our situation. He promised he would do his best to get one from another store and give us a call when it came in. I had to come up with something like a bed rail until then. After Christina was in bed, I put two chairs with the back to the edge of the bed, then a large wicker blanket chest next to it, and a small foot stool wedged between the wall and the chest. It could not move. The next morning while she was still sleeping, I removed them all until the next night. Two days later, we got a call that the bed rail was in. We picked it up and expressed our appreciation to the store manager. You get a good feeling when people care and help.

Christina had only two major so-called "accidents" in the many years I cared for her at our home. We had a soft plastic cover over our mattress for years. It paid off. Once I woke up and felt that the sheet between my wife and me was wet. I was confused and surprised. I turned the light on in our bathroom, got a fresh nightgown and underwear, and one fitted sheet and a top sheet. I said to her, "I have to put another nightgown on you." After that was done, I put her in a chair with armrests and put the bed blanket around her. The next part was pulling the sheets off and replacing them with clean ones. Then I put her back in bed and pulled the sheet over her and then put the blanket back on. She fell asleep quickly.

Before our afternoon walk, I brought her to the bathroom and left her there for a short time. When I came back, she was standing. I could see the soft stool going down her legs into her slacks and shoes. How was I to start cleaning her? I used a whole roll of toilet paper and wiped as much off as I could while she was still standing. Using moist towelettes, I cleaned her buttocks and legs, cleaned the toilet seat, and let her sit down. I put all the soiled clothes in the basin of the vanity, including her shoes, which I later put in a plastic bag and threw in the garbage. I cleaned the floor, washed my hands, and led her into the bedroom where I dressed her. We did not walk that afternoon.

These changes came unexpectedly, and since I did not know what else might happen, I called the Office of Aging and explained our situation. I asked for help and was told a case worker would be assigned to assess our conditions at home.

This would be the first time in our lives that we had to deal with a government agency to help us. A social worker phoned and made an appointment. When he arrived, I explained our situation to him again and said we need help right now, not only with bathing but also with my wife's diet. His answer was, "Use a cookbook." My reply was, "Cookbooks are for people who are not ill. This is a special illness; she needs a dietician who has the training and experience to prepare a diet for her."

He explained that we had to fill out a form called a "Discretionary Income Worksheet." We mailed this in to the Office of Aging, and later we did get a letter telling us that we were put on a waiting list.

I called a private nursing company. They came out the next day. The nurse came early in the morning and tried to wash my wife's face first, but Christina did not let her do it. It could be that there was not the right chemistry or the nurse did not have experience with Alzheimer's patients. When I saw how she was upsetting my wife, I told her to stop trying. She asked if she could come back the next day, but I said, "No."

Close to our home in a very small shopping center, I noticed there was a hair salon. We stopped and went in and I explained to the manager about my wife's illness and asked if she could help us. She replied that there were no openings and she closed at 4:00 p.m. The disappointment must have been visible on my face as we walked toward the door past all the chairs filled with people. Then one of the beauticians who had heard our conversation walked toward us and said, "I will do her hair." A load fell off my shoulders. When it was my wife's turn, the stylist told me that her grandmother had had Alzheimer's and the family had taken care of her. She knew what it meant. She was a very compassionate person. My wife must have sensed this and the two got along well. She made appointments for Christina for the next four weeks.

One Saturday when we parked our car for the weekly visit to the hair dresser, I opened the door to let her out. I said, "It is time to do your hair." She did not move, so I came closer and gave her a hand and put my arm around her back and said, "The nice lady is waiting for you to do your hair." She did not get out of the car.

The beautician always came to the waiting area and walked her to the chair to wash her hair. That day, the shampoo was not the problem. It was the rinsing that upset Christina. She always had to bend her head backward, but this time it triggered some fear. When she was sitting under the dryer she walked away from it. That happened only once. From that day on, going to do her hair was no longer a pleasure trip.

Every Saturday morning, she became restless during the rinsing, and it made me nervous too. I was as scared and upset as she was. What else could I do? I could not wash her hair at home. I found out that there was a shampoo that did not need water or rinsing. I tried it on myself, but I did not feel refreshed and clean, so that did not work. When Saturday morning came, I would park each time in a different location. Christina would walk to the shop and sit down in the waiting area with no problem. But when it came to the rinse, one person could not handle her. She needed an extra person to keep her head backward, and that was the way it was done from then on.

One Saturday, the beautician told me that she was moving somewhere else to start a new life. It was a shock. Most people who lived in this area lived and died here and did not travel much in their lives. About a year later, we got a letter from her. She was happy and thanked us for being there at the time she needed a change and new direction in her life.

One of the many things you need to do when you move from one state to another is to find a medical doctor. The last time, it was easy, as there were doctors in our church in Louisville. So we started asking, "Do you know a good doctor?" Sometimes we did not get much of an answer, until one person said, "Why don't you ask Rose? She is a registered nurse and works for a doctor." We did and made an appointment.

My wife could not answer the questions or undress and dress herself, so we stayed together during our hour-long physical. I am quite sure doctors do not like to have two people in their office or examination room. However, this doctor did not seem to mind. We were physically both in good shape, except for my wife's dementia and her blood pressure, which was high. We had to come back to have it rechecked, and on the third visit, medication was prescribed. Christina had always taken aspirin as prevention, so I did not expect any problems. She did not want to take the blood pressure pill, so I had to go to the drug store and buy a pill crusher. Applesauce and the crushed pill did the trick.

Our son came to visit us. We talked about the respite, which we received free, and suddenly he said, "Dad, why don't you go out to your shopping center and I will take care of Ma. You need a break." It seemed to me a good idea. I did not have any problem with it, because my wife and son were very close.

I drove on my favorite highway to the shopping center and this time, I really enjoyed it. Before I knew it, it was time for the trip home. From the shopping center, you had to take a few exit roads to get back on the highway. Suddenly, I got a strange fearful idea in my head. I was afraid that my wife was in the hospital. Why? I did not know. How could it be? Our son was with her. What could have happened to her? I tried to push it out of my mind. I turned the radio on, but the feeling did not go away; that inexplicable fear that she was in the hospital stayed with me. A soundless voice continued inside me, and it came back again and again. *Was I making up a fact that was not true? Was I dreaming while I was driving?* When I came to our street, I was relieved to see our son's car parked in front of the house. I drove the car into the driveway and into the garage and said to myself, *See? You were wrong. She is still at home. You worked yourself up for nothing.* I opened the door and said, "I am home." No answer. I looked in the living room and the bedroom, and no one was at home. So I said to myself, *They are out for a walk* and sat down in the kitchen. There was a piece of paper on the counter top. The short note was, "I had to call 911. Ma went to the hospital."

I took off and drove to the community hospital in the next town. The country roads were deserted most of the time, so I made good time. At the desk I asked for my wife who had just been admitted, and I was directed to the emergency room, where I found our son with my wife. She was hooked up to a machine which recorded her blood pressure and heart rate, neither of which was stable. Our son told me what had happen. He was in the living room and Christina was walking and ended up in the bedroom, where she stayed for some time. He heard her scream a loud and painful sound. He rushed to the room and found her lying on the bed. After that, she did not move and was very pale. He talked to her, but there was no reaction. He took precautions to be sure she could not roll off the bed and went to the next room and called 911. The phone cord was long enough so he could keep an eye on her. It did not take long for the ambulance to arrive at our home. After checking her vital signs, they called for a life support unit to meet them halfway up the road to the hospital. Our son was in the ambulance. The hospital must have called our doctor to get more information. When I asked, "What is wrong with her?" I did not get a good answer. A doctor came and told us that she would be admitted and would be transferred to a room. After waiting some time, we were allowed to see her in her room. We stayed with her for quite some time. When visiting hours were over, we tried once more to get information. But the nurse said, "The doctor was called away and will be in tomorrow." We were suspicious, but what could we do if the professionals were dodging our questions?

The next day, I went to the hospital and found her sitting in a chair with a dull expression in her eyes. I was very upset and went to the nurses' station and asked, "Why is she not in her bed, but sitting in a chair?" The nurse went with me to her room and said, "We had to do this because we could not keep her in bed. It was for her own safety, so she would hurt not herself." I could see that she needed cleaning. If this hospital could not keep her in bed, at least they could keep her clean. I immediately insisted she be cleaned. She was not the same person I had left behind, yesterday, at home. Did the doctor or nurses know that she had dementia? My son and I had told them. The doctor was not in that day and no further information was given. She had high blood pressure and unstable vital signs, but no one would tell us what they were doing or what medication she had received. The next day, I came in her room, and there she was still sitting in the chair. This time, the soft stool was dripping from her seat to the floor. I went to the nurses' station and said, "Clean her up and dress her. She is leaving this hospital right now." We had to wait some time. The nurse came back with papers and told us that the hospital doctor had called our doctor and the high-blood-pressure pills were not needed any more. I was not only upset but very angry. She had taken high-blood-pressure medication for years and apparently there had been no need for it. It was a miracle that she was still alive. Now she had to take another medication to keep her calm. She was always a very quiet and happy person. The hospital portrayed her as a violent person when they restrained her in her chair. The staff did know that she had dementia. Most doctors did not know about this illness except from their textbooks and were not trained to diagnose the illness properly. This hospital had done a very bad job of treating her. Could it be that when she was in bed she wanted to go to the bathroom? She could not speak or indicate with signs what she wanted. Her routine was interrupted, but her needs stayed the same and were ignored by the staff, who wrongly labeled her condition. This, on top of the wrong medication she had used for many years, had certainly done damage.

The next day, we returned to our normal routine. While she was standing outside the tub to be washed and dried, I noticed a small open sore. I dried it off very carefully and put zinc oxide on it. I covered it with a piece of gauze and taped it in place. This upset me. Hospitals have a bad track record for open sores. This was my first experience. By keeping it dry and applying zinc oxide, I thought it should heal pretty fast. She had always been a fast healer. This was another disappointment. The next problem was that she lost control over her bladder and bowel movements.

With careful planning, I could keep her as regular as possible, but that was my intervention, not her ability to control her urges. Her sleeping patterns became erratic as well. Many times she would just wake up in the middle of the night and sit up in bed. With gentle urging, she would lie down again. I was a light sleeper, so I always knew when she woke up.

In the mornings, I poured her a cup of tea and prepared one slice of bread. I removed the crusts and cut it in quarters because she was not wearing her lower partial plate. At first, she remained at the table. After she ate the first piece of bread, she stood up and walked away. I followed her with the plate in my hands. When she was done with that piece, I would give her another one until she had eaten one slice of bread. That was all she ate. If her tea got cold, I would give her fresh hot tea when she sat down again. Bathing had changed, too. If she did not want to go in the bathroom, I tried again later, and if she had not changed her mind, I let it go to until the next day.

The Office of Aging still had us on the waiting list. I called and explained how the situation had changed and requested to get some help now. We were told we had moved up on the list, but due to cuts in social benefits, we still had to wait. I asked a retired registered nurse at our church if she would help wash Christina in the morning. She agreed to try. She came and talked to her and slowly tried to wash her face. She knew from experience this was difficult, as my wife refused to let her wash. She knew that pushing it would not go anywhere and explained this to me about dementia patients. She stayed for a while and did not mind trying to communicate with my wife in a quiet and loving way. Knowing this, I did not mind that the Office of Aging could not help us. Could they have done better? We will never know.

Our children, pastor, and doctor had told me, "You have done your best. It is time to step back and let others do it for you now." I knew that someday this would happen, but not yet. I wanted to take care of her as long as I could, even if it meant that it would not get any better. I truly believed that I could better care for her at home. When it comes to matters of the heart, common sense is not present. When our daughters were in high school, they worked part time in a local nursing home and told me, "Never go as a patient to a nursing home." I had not dismissed the possibility that it might happen and filled out applications for three nursing homes which had an Alzheimer's unit. Every year I received a letter from these homes asking if we still wanted to stay on the waiting list. My answer was always yes, and I kept a copy of my reply.

After her return from the hospital, we did not walk for two days. But we started again. One day we were almost home when suddenly I felt her leaning on my right arm so heavily that it felt as if she was falling into a hole and hanging onto me. We stopped and I don't remember how long we stood like that, until I felt that the pressure was gone and we walked home slowly. It was only about a hundred feet. I called the doctor and I was told he would call me back. When he did, I told him what had happen to us. He responded that it was a mini-stroke or TIA, which stands for transient ischemic attack. They last a few minutes and nothing can be done about them. The walks had to end, which ended the benefit of exercise as well.

Our pastor was well aware of our problem, and he set the wheels in motion to get the women of our church involved in helping. I signed up for Meals on Wheels and we received the meal around noon time. I took a portion for her and put it in the small mixer we had bought for her meals. This was not new, but part of the preparations to feed her in the past. She responded. I could feed her again. Although the amount she ate was very small, at least there was some change. One day during Christina's meal, as I was waiting until all the food had cleared her mouth and was swallowed, she suddenly said, as clear as a bell, "You are a good husband." She had not spoken in a long time. I got a strange feeling in me and tears came to my eyes, and I hugged her and said, "You are the best, I love you so much."

It was a statement from her to me, expressing her appreciation that I cared for her no matter what the conditions were. She had taken care of me and our whole family so unselfishly without any complaint for so many years, often in difficult circumstances. Now it was my turn to be the caregiver, and I did it with the same dedication she had shown me for all those years.

Many men walk away from situations like this when the domestic and sex services are no longer provided. Society accepts this as they do so many wrongful practices.

Our daughter Karen flew out to visit us. Her brother picked her up from the airport. Both of them were shocked to see how much weight Christina had lost and the change in her facial expressions. We talked for quite some time, not ignoring her, and they advised me to start looking for placement in a nursing home.

CHAPTER SEVEN

Making Tough Choices

Our daughter made an appointment at one of the nursing homes where we were on the waiting list. During our visit, our son would watch Christina.

The director of admissions received us and told us about the facility. However, she would not let us visit the Alzheimer's unit. We were impressed with the general conditions and atmosphere of this home. Since my wife was already on the waiting list, the director told us that in case of an urgent need, some arrangements could be made. A doctor's affidavit would be most helpful in finding a bed for her at a shorter notice. However, we were disappointed that we were not allowed to see the Alzheimer's unit.

Our son and daughter had left to visit their younger sister Ellen and her family in New Jersey. When Karen returned, she was shocked to see how her mother had changed for the worse in such a short time. She said to me, "Dad, you better get help for Ma; you can't keep this up. It is not good for the either of you."

The days and nights came and went. There was no improvement. I did not increase the doses of medication as advised, because I was suspicious of this advice. Sometimes Christina accepted food. The long nights and interruptions of sleep was a drain on both of us. When Christina woke up during the night, she sat up in bed and did not move for a while. Initially I would sit up with her, but I could not do that for long as it was an uncomfortable position. I would lie down and hold her hand. When she finally put her head down and went to sleep, I was too upset to relax and do the same. I could not fall back to sleep.

When she woke up again, we started all over. Usually after the second interruption, she slept until daylight and stayed in bed for some time. I prepared breakfast and gave it to her in bed as I used to do on Saturdays and Sundays back when I still worked and was looking forward to retirement.

When she did not open her lips to accept food, I would try juice. I held the glass in my hands to let her drink the orange juice, which she accepted. I would prop her up with pillows behind her back to make her comfortable, but I soon realized this was a thing of the past and would not be safe in her current condition. I let her stay in bed in the morning until she had to go to the bathroom. We ate our other meals in the kitchen. I covered the table with a large piece of clear plastic so that any spills could be easily wiped off. It turned out that I was the one who did most of the spilling. Many times, it would spill all over the walls. We were making a mess. A carpenter was willing to install wainscoting—forty-inch-high oak slats, the same kind as our kitchen cabinets, from the opening of the dining room to the hallway. After the carpenter was finished, I covered the nail holes with soft oak wood filling and took the small electrical sander and made the surface as smooth as silk. The first coat of clear varnish soaked in quickly. The second was applied the same day. Two days later, the final coat. It broke the monotonous routine for a short time and we had solved one small problem, of which I was the main offender.

In the afternoon when the sun was at the back of our home, we did not use the patio. We had an umbrella that we could angle to catch the sunrays and create a shady location around the table, but we found a better place in the afternoon. We opened the small garage door in the back and the big one in the front. The sun cast a shadow on the driveway, which took the heat away, and a breeze flowed through the garage. We put two chairs with a small table in between but very close to the edge of the concrete floor. I made tea and brought out cookies in a metal container.

We would watch the cows across the street. They were always behind the last two homes at the dead end of the street. Traffic was sparse at that time, and no one walked at that time of the day. It was an American *siesta* time, which the two of us used to relax. The cows were not too close to our home, and I was happy about that because I can't stand flies. Even so, I hung two old-fashioned fly catchers in our garage, the small, round cardboard containers with a spiral strip coated with very sticky glue. We did not catch too many flies in our garage.

During the day, my mind was always asking, *What am I going to do to prepare her for the big change? Should I tell her or not? Would she understand what I told her?* It would be the first time in our lives that we would be separated. I did not want to let her go. It would mean others who did not have the same love and dedication would take over my responsibilities. I also remembered what our daughters had told us: "Never go into a nursing home." Her short stay in the hospital was another reminder. How could trained medical personnel neglect a patient and in essence do harm, whether intended or not?

As days went by, there was no change in her. I decided to call our doctor and explain to him what we had to go through each day and night. He also knew that I had taken care of her for more than five years and that according to our children, it was time to let her go. They said they did not want to lose two parents. I told him what the director of admissions had told me, that a placement recommended by a doctor would help.

Within a week, I got a call from the nursing home and was told that a day was set for admitting her. It still left me another ten days to prepare both of us for this. I called our son and asked him if he would come to assist me with this emotional and depressing task. He agreed to be there for me and his mother.

Most of that day I spent rehearsing what I would say to my wife. I decided to tell her that she was not feeling well and was not sleeping at night. She was losing weight and was not that active anymore, rarely walking or going out. My mind told me, *This is not right. You are only recording facts, hiding your real feelings of letting her go.* It is not easy to put into words your feelings and compassion. So I tried again and again, gave up for some time, and then started all over. It seemed that my mind had become an empty space. Talking had never been my best side. I did not like small talk. I knew I would be a very bad salesperson. I remember one statement, "Conciseness marks the master." It is a lost art in our society, where a stream of words seems to be the rule, and in this stream the meaning is lost. We use a lot of words but say nothing. The question *What should I tell her, or should I just take her?* was in my mind every moment. It would be the first time in our long married life that we would be separated. I also thought what being separated meant in our society. No matter how separations come, from a divorce or another way, such as bringing a loved one to a nursing home, they brought with them a stigma. I felt the stigma of not being able to care for her anymore in a special way. The staff at the facility had their training, but it was and always would be a job that had to be done, like any other job with its ups and downs.

This would be especially true in my wife's case, with the understanding of Alzheimer's still in its infancy. I did not have training, but on the other hand, I had the compassion, the time, and the love, as well as support and instructions from the support group. Would she be able to understand what it would mean to leave her home and enter a strange place where she would not see me every minute of the day and night? What if she woke up and missed the comfort of being held in her time of need?

There is no doubt that her new surroundings would be a big shock to her. For me, it would also be a great shock not to have her around, not be able to care for her as I had done for more than five years. I would miss her company and her personality, which had not changed. These questions did not stop, but went on in my mind every day. At night, I did get the sleep to renew me for the next day. The nights were not the normal ones, but I knew I had to get my deep sleep to go on the next day and the days after that. When you are in a situation like this, your common sense and clear thinking do not work the way they should. Emotions and fear get the upper hand. I decided to solve one of the problems by calling our daughter. I was sure she could help her father now and give him advice.

She knew what was going on. She had seen it herself, so no explanation was needed. I asked, "Should I tell Ma what I am going to do?" In the past, we did not make any decisions without communicating with each other.

Her reply was, "Pa, it is still better to tell her, even when she does not understand or comprehend the meaning of your words. You will have the peace of mind that you did it. You are not in control of her mind. The advancement of her illness goes on. How far gone is it? We will know to a certain extent by how she reacts, if she has any reaction at all. You have taken care of her at home for more than five years, which had deprived both of you from the pleasures of a well-deserved retirement. You both worked and raised us. You will never regret telling her about going to a nursing home. It is good for your peace of mind."

When we traveled by plane abroad or to our children, I had made out a standard list of items for each of us to take on our trip. It covered almost anything to be included in our luggage. If we did not need an item, we took it off the list. This came in handy now. I prepared a list for the nursing home, but it was also very sad, as it would be the last one I wrote for her. I assumed that the clothes she would wear would be the same as in our home. I was also told that she would go out once a week on a trip with other patients, so I had to include a raincoat and a winter coat with gloves and a scarf. All of this had to be labeled with her name and room number after admission. I postponed telling her about the nursing home until the day before the trip in case she forgot about it. This happened when I told her things too far ahead of time. Later I found out that my rationale was not right. I assumed that we were dealing as equals, an understanding which did not exist anymore, but through the years was an established rule. I did not accept her as a dementia patient but as my wife. I had known for almost seventy years; you do not turn this off in a short time.

Professional persons call this denial, and of course it is, but they seem to say that denial is a result of an illness. However, denial is also a part of our life. It starts early in life, but we do not call it by that name. If a small child does something wrong, he or she will blame somebody or something else for it. This denial goes on into adulthood. If a marriage goes wrong, one spouse blames the other. There is a lot of denial associated with dementia. Compare the difference between how we treat people with cancer or heart problems. Research for these two diseases far exceeds research for Alzheimer's.

I would only be caring for Christina at home for one more day. I remember that day well. Christina was sitting in her favorite chair. I pulled up a chair to sit close to her and held her hand and said, "You know, we are now retired for five years and we have lived in this house all those years. I have taken care of you to the best of my ability. We became members of the senior citizens group—not one, but two. We went on trips with them and on our own. We visited our children and when we had to fly, I gave you medication to prevent you from having motion sickness. You had to take this before you went on the plane and it seemed to work for you. We came back from the visits and walked and shopped in the malls, one of your favorite pastimes. We went grocery shopping and went to church. I know you could not sing the hymns, but we always shared the hymnal. The members of the church were friendly to you. Our pastor is one of the most caring persons we know. He backed up his words with actions to do all he could, not only for you but all the other Alzheimer's patients, too.

"When you were in the hospital, the doctors soon found out what you had, but did not tell us. They just told me that the medication you had taken was no longer necessary. The staff of the hospital apparently had never taken care of an Alzheimer's patient. This lack of knowledge made them behave badly. This was the second time you received the wrong treatment in the same hospital. You had to take another medication you might not need and it caused you to get confused at night, so you woke up, something you had never done as long as we were married. You used to be a very sound sleeper. We did not get help from the Office of Aging, but were put on a waiting list. They did not give us any help in getting a diet for you.

"However, the doctor in this nursing home knows a lot more about your illness. He is in charge of this unit. He seems to be a nice and caring person. I feel comfortable with him. We will go to the nursing home. He will examine you and you will stay there. It is not easy for me to do this, but our son will come tonight and help me. Right now I am overwhelmed with fear and uncertainty about you and me. I love you very much. You have lost too much weight, and it is not you. You have changed. It could be that new medication, but I will be there every day to visit you in the nursing home."

She looked at me and said, "That is nice." When she responded like that, I knew that she could not have comprehended all that I had told her. Maybe the last part was reassuring to her. So I tried to tell her again in a much shorter way, but she did not respond at all. I hugged her and kissed her and said again, "I will visit you in the nursing home every day," and held her in my arms.

I do not remember when our son arrived that afternoon or the time we spent together that evening. I know that I must have washed and dressed her, but the memory is foggy. I don't remember whose car we drove to the nursing home. We must have had breakfast, but that is also lost. I do not remember getting in the car or if we were sitting together in the back. The only thing that I remember was at the door of the nursing home, letting her get in first. I do not remember who took her to the doctor. I remember sitting with our son in the office of the director of admissions. She was a registered nurse who had spent the last years of her profession in the nursing-home industry. What we talked about is covered in darkness. The next thing I remembered was that we were in the Alzheimer's unit looking out the window; then my emotions became too strong and I started to cry.

Before we left the facility, we went to the office of the medical director. He was a friendly white-haired man. He greeted us and said, "This is the first patient I have examined and admitted to the Alzheimer's unit in such a very advanced stage. I will be taking her off the medication in about a week." The last sentence confirmed my suspicion. I said to myself, *You were right. This is now the second time that she has received medication that was not necessary, and it did more harm than good.* It certainly did mental harm to me as well as the physical harm it did to my wife, but we will never know. *Are the two doctors who gave her those medications sales people for the pharmaceutical industry rather than doctors?* From that moment I became very careful about prescriptions written for her.

We are the greatest drug users in the world. Almost every American is on drugs—not one, but several. We love to take them; it is a national addiction. The pharmaceutical industry benefits from this. They charge their own citizens more money for the identical drug made in the United States but sold overseas. I still remember at our senior citizens' group meeting when a representative of a drug company came to talk about drugs and asked, "Who is taking medication?" Almost everyone raised their hand.

The doctor showed me a chart with the seven stages of Alzheimer's. Number six and seven pertained to Christina, with the exception that she could control her bowel and bladder movements, with my help. She was in the last phase of stage six. She could only speak a few words. The last part of stage seven was the terminal stage of Alzheimer's disease.

My son and I left the building and got in the car, but where we went and what we did that day is deeply buried in my mind. I have no memory at all. All I remember was that the director of admissions and the case worker had told me in previous meetings that there was no restriction on visiting hours, which were posted on the walls but not enforced. In fact, they had told me that I could come in at any time.

So I said to our son, "Let us test if what they told us is true." It was dark; we parked the car and rang the doorbell. It took sometime before a security guard came and opened the door. I said, "We would like to see my wife, who was admitted today." He came up with excuses; the first one was that visiting hours were over and they did not allow visitors in after visiting hours. I cut him off and told him that the director of admissions had told us we could come in at any time. He called the supervisor, who took some time before he showed up. I repeated the same request, with the statement from the director and the case worker. He did not say much but allowed us to go in and see my wife. Our son stayed in the lobby. I went to her floor. I introduced myself. The staff had received a phone call that I was coming. I found her room. I just wanted to look at her.

I walked quietly into the room and found her asleep. I was happy she was not awake or sitting up. I kissed her on the forehead and left. I was very fortunate and grateful to our son, who had offered to be there with me on this very difficult day. I knew it was not easy for him. I will always remember this support given by him in the darkest moment of our lives.

I had given up the care of my wife to others. She had moved out, not of her free will or as a result of problems between us, but because of the problems of providing care for her at home and wrongful medications. The house was empty. When I arrived home, there was no one to welcome me, to kiss and talk to, no coffee smell or smell of a dinner being prepared. No domestic activities. It was a house without life. Her spirit was still around. It showed in the paintings and pictures on the wall. She had arranged the room by placing furniture in such a way as to make the room look larger. Curtains and drapes hung in the living room and dining room. In other rooms, Venetian blinds hung and there was a selection of brass lamps and antiques from the old country, which had been made and used by our relatives. The European crystal stood safe behind doors in a corner curio cabinet. Other more precious art items were stored in a cabinet with four glass doors and three glass shelves. The house was like a music box whose chimes did not play anymore.

CHAPTER EIGHT

Alzheimer's Unit

The next morning, I left to visit my wife in the nursing home. It was quite a change not only for me, but for her. The normal routine was gone. I do not know who fed her that first morning, but I was sure she felt the difference. She was not sitting in her familiar chair at the kitchen table and taking a slice from her plate. I did not have the faintest idea how breakfast or any other meal was served in this place. She would be sitting somewhere and someone would be feeding her in a way she was not accustomed to. There would be a different voice and someone trying to keep her from walking away, which only had to do with her illness and nothing else.

She was not able to express herself, but she felt the change in surroundings and the many persons who were around her. I had given the staff detailed information about her daily activities, but it was put in a file. Maybe it was smiled at with the idea, "We do it differently here."

When I came to the floor, I went to the charge nurse. She was friendly and listened to what I told her about my wife. The nurses not only gave bed care, but had the time to comfort the patients by talking. All of us know that a friendly and understanding nurse can give a depressed patient just what they need at that moment. You cannot put this in a job description, but if there is enough staff, it can be done.

After our conversation with the charge nurse, I went to Christina's room but she was not there. She was not in the hallway, either. So I went across to the other hall and there she was, walking away toward the opposite end. I sped up and caught up with her, slowed down and took her hand. She turned slowly, and there was only a slight sign of recognition. Even calling her name did not change much, so we walked together as we had done in our neighborhood. We walked up and down the hall and then across to the other side, walked that hall and then back across, walking that hall up and down until we came to the end. There was a table with two chairs and I guided her into one and pulled the other up close to her, holding her hand and looking at her. There was that faraway look in her eyes. Talking to her and calling her name did not make any difference, but I kept holding her hands and stroking them. It did not have any obvious effect, but I knew that even if she did not react, the feeling would never leave her. It would always be there, no matter what happened. She was utterly confused, and she could not express herself. She seemed so lonely. When it was time to leave, I just kissed her and said, "I'll be back."

I knew she could not talk anymore, but she knew my voice. She felt my hand and her female intuition told her that I would be there for her. My voice and touch would be our only way of communicating from now on.

When I returned in the afternoon, she was walking again. It was quite different from the morning. It was very crowded. Patients were walking or sitting everywhere. It looked like downtown New York at lunchtime. I met the charge nurse, who was a male. From the first moment I saw Danny, I liked him. He was friendly and introduced himself. We had a short talk because he was busy handing out medication and keeping an eye on some of those who needed constant attention. Most of them congregated in front of the nurses' station and in the dayroom. The hall was less crowded, and that was the place where we were heading. We walked slowly. I held Christina's hand up and down the hall from one end to the other. When we changed to another hall, I stayed very close to her to protect her from people who might bump into her. Once in the other hall, we were relatively safe from bumping into other patients, who were male and resided on that side. We walked for quite a while, and then we returned to the women's side, where we rested at the end of the hall.

While we were resting, I heard over the P.A. system, "Trays are up." This was to alert personnel who were working in the rooms to finish what they were doing and come and help with the distribution of food and also help with the patients who needed feeding. I said to my wife, "Let us see how this works." I helped her.

We walked down the hall to the nurses' station. There was a cart holding ten trays on each side. Each had cups with lids, fruit, cartons with milk, and juices. Each tray had a card with a name on it. The staff was already there to bring the trays to each person, and they removed the lids to tell the patients what was in each cup. If the patient had tea or coffee, they asked if they wanted sugar or milk. They took the fork, knife, and spoon out of the waxed-paper envelope. I asked, "Is my wife's tray on the cart?" The answer was, "Probably no; it goes by alphabetical order."

"How many more carts are coming?" I asked.

"Two more."

We waited ten minutes and another cart came up. We checked. No tray for Christina. The staff said it would be on the last one. I said, "If this takes another ten minutes, it will be late and I want to feed her. How can we change this?" I was told, "You have to talk to the charge nurse on the seven-to-three shift." So we waited till the last cart came up.

Christina and I continued to walk and saw some residents sitting in what were called Geri chairs. They were used to restrain patients and also for feeding. But after that was done, patients remained in the chairs for quite some time. The reason given for this was to protect them from hurting themselves. There was some truth in this, but it was also easier for the staff. To let them walk would require more personnel. Nursing home managers are experts at making up reasons to downplay the permanent shortage of nursing aids and other personnel. On this floor, there were too many people walking in all directions, and they stayed in the same small area. The easiest way to reduce this number was to put some patients in the Geri chairs. These Geri chairs gave a cheap impression and were very uncomfortable to stay in for a long time. It reminded me of the old baby high chairs, the ones where you pulled out the tray and lifted the baby from the floor and guided her feet and body in such a way that the feet were under the tray and she sat on the wooden seat. The same principle was used here, except the babies were now mature adults. Under the tray were two chrome pipes that fitted into a smaller chrome pipe under each arm rest. One side served as the hinge and the other had a push-and-pull pin which fitted into the holes to adjust for the size of the person who would sit in the chair.

The staff showed me how to use this chair. I put my wife in it. It did not feel right to see her in that kind of chair. I did not restrain her at home. It upset me. Here she sat like a small child. She could not get out it if she wanted to. Her freedom was taken away from her. She now depended on a person who did not know her. The staff had their own rules. The tray was brought to her and put in front of her. I removed the lids off the containers and saw the food. One was soup. She did not like soup, so I did not give that to her. I saw a milk carton and she never drank milk. There were mashed potatoes and vegetables, which I put on the plate and then went to a table where there was a pitcher with gravy. I poured some over it and went back to feed her. She did not eat much, but drank some of the orange juice. When she did not want to eat anymore, I pulled the pin, flipped the tray over to the other side of the chair, and helped her out. We walked again. I put the tray back on the chair and told the staff that she did not want to eat anymore. It was now almost three hours since I had come, and it was time for me to go home and eat. While we were walking I said, "I am going home to eat, but I will be back every morning and afternoon each day of the year," and kissed her. She did not react and kept on walking.

The next morning, I saw her walking when I came from the elevator. I took her by the hand and said, "I am here." No reply. We kept on walking, and when we passed the nurses' station, the charge nurse was there, and we stopped.

"Good morning; do you have a moment?" I asked.

"Yes," she replied.

"Yesterday afternoon I was here and stayed to feed her. I noticed on her tray a carton of milk, but she does not like milk. She never drank it at home, but she does like yogurt. Could you please make this change in her menu?"

"I will give this information to the social worker."

"The social worker has received a sheet with information about what she likes to eat, her toileting habits, and her daily routines."

"I will remind her; it might take some time."

"I also noticed that her tray comes on the last cart. I will be feeding her from now on in the afternoon, and I was told by your staff that you can ask to have her tray placed on the first cart. There is a long time between the arrival of the first cart and the last one. Can you help me?"

"The kitchen and dietary staff will have to make that change. I will call them about this."

"Thank you very much."

While we walked, I looked into the rooms and saw that most of them were empty. When we went to the other side, which had more men and only a few women, it was quite different. Most men were still in their beds. At the end of the hall was a man sitting in a good chair. He had a white shirt and tie, and his white hair was combed. As soon as he noticed us, he began to say, "Help me, help me, help me, help me." We stopped in front of him and I asked, "What can we do for you?" He looked at us for some time, but he did not answer. I asked him again, but he kept quiet and seemed content that somebody paid attention to him. I asked more questions, but no reply. It seemed that all he wanted was to have somebody close by him who showed some compassion and interest. We stayed with him for a while and I said, "My wife and I will visit you again." Then we turned around and walked slowly away. He kept quiet. The charge nurse told me that my wife would go on a bus trip with some of the other patients. This would always be on a Tuesday.

In the afternoon, I found Christina sitting in one of those terrible, uncomfortable Geri chairs. I took her out of that chair. The nurse said, "She looked tired, so we let her rest."

We did our usual walk along the hallways.

Before we knew it, the first cart with trays had arrived on the floor. It took some time before my wife's tray came up. In the meantime, we found a nice, quiet spot far away from the others, and I asked the staff to bring the tray to our table, which they gladly did because I was doing part of their job. Her appetite was not good. I gave her only the food I knew she liked, but I also tried some of the others, even the soup that she never ate. I made it a habit to try one spoonful of whatever was on the tray. All containers with food had lids. There was also a milk carton. I had given the staff detailed instructions about what she liked to eat. Milk was not on that list, but ice cream and yogurt were.

The next morning, I again told the charge nurse that Christina did not like milk. It took some time before it was removed from her menu. If it was there, I did not open the milk carton, but left it on the tray. Yogurt was an item that was not given to anybody at that time. It had to be ordered. It was the small eight-ounce container.

It was a depressing feeling to be there with her, even more so when I had to leave her in this place where everybody was a stranger. I talked to her, but there was no response of eye movement or turning of her head. I had no idea how long it would take for her to get back to the condition she had been at home. She missed the constant feeling of love and care. The surroundings were also different. There was no yard to look at. She missed her favorite chair in which she drank her tea or coffee. At this time of year, we were always watching the farmer harvesting his corn and then preparing his fields for the spring.

In the afternoon, I did not see Danny, the charge nurse. I felt secure when he was on duty. He could handle a particular patient, Henry, who was extremely strong and had unexpected violent outbursts. When these outbursts occurred, someone usually got hurt or fell. If a report was written, it said, "Patient fell." The victim was mentioned, but never the one who caused this accident. In the nursing-home industry, it was a well-known fact that patients in Alzheimer's units often fell. I had this with my wife at home, too. However, this fact is used to cover up other cases where it is the fault not of the victim but of inadequate staffing. If you are only an occasional visitor, you do not know about these things.

The perpetrator seemed to have an unusual shield of protection, which was unfair but also dangerous to the other patients. Henry could not walk and was restricted to a wheelchair. His hands were dangerous and very fast. He had learned to maneuver his chair very well. If Henry had one of his outbursts and was reported, Danny was always very quick to respond and always approached him from the back. First Danny tried to pull him backward to his room, and if that did not work, he just moved Henry away from the other patients. The staff kept Henry separated from the others. Danny went to his medicine cart and gave him a shot, which calmed him down, and then took him to his room. I did not understand why the management allowed this person to be in the Alzheimer's unit. It was clearly stated in the agreement that if a patient harmed himself or others, he could be removed from the institution.

We would chat with Danny frequently when he was doing his medication rounds. He would talk about the working conditions on this floor, but also about the many residents who did not get any visits from family or relatives. We also shared some personal information. One day, he told me that his father had cancer. He did not go into details and I did not asked what kind of cancer it was. Several weeks later, the staff brought a newspaper in which the passing of Danny's father was announced with information about the final services. I went to the afternoon wake. I met his mother and brothers and expressed our condolences to the family.

One morning, a woman came out of her room naked and walked down the hall. She did not pay any attention to us but kept walking until she reached the nursing station. The excited staff quickly tried to cover her with an eight-by-eleven piece of paper, which did not cover much, so they had to go to a linen cart and pull a sheet off to cover her and bring her back to her room to be dressed again. She did not resist, but went back to her room. The staff told me, "This is not the first time," and they were right. The next time it happened, she was combative and resistant. Sometimes, after she was dressed, she was put in a Geri chair with the tray as close to her body as possible. She was also an escape artist. She worked on getting out of her chair for a long time. As we walked up and down the hall, she did not give up. On a return walk, I saw her sliding under the tray and out of the chair. Sometimes the staff used a long-sleeved top to restrict her hand movements, but this did not work either. Even when she did not have the urge to walk naked, she always walked by herself. We passed her quite a few times on our walks up and down the hall. One time she stopped and said, "I like you." Other times, she walked alongside us and I held her hand, but not for long. Then she walked on her own again.

It took a long time before my wife started to eat a little better. This made the afternoon visit more pleasant. I had the time to check her bowel movements, which had been like clockwork at home, but not here. I had to check in private, and I found a way. There were several unoccupied rooms. These rooms gave me the opportunity to check her by touching her slacks. If I found a bowel movement, I took Christina to a nurses' aide and asked her to change and clean her.

"Is it small, medium, or large?"

"What do you mean by that? I don't know what is small, medium, or large. She needs to be cleaned and changed."

"I will be back in a minute."

The time went ticking by, but no one showed up to change my wife. I was very upset and said to myself, *How would you feel if this happened to you? What would she do if this happened to her children at home?* It is embarrassing, especially for an older adult who cannot control her bodily functions anymore. At home, she was used to a regular routine. My wife could not ask anymore, and this was not her fault. So I tried another nurses' aide. She helped right away, and I expressed my appreciation. "I have little ones at home and I treat my people here the same as I do my children at home," she said.

CHAPTER NINE

Asking for Help

It was early November and the nursing-home staff asked me if I wanted to help serve the Thanksgiving meal. I put my name on the list. No one else signed up for this occasion of happiness and thanks. There was still time. I talked to my pastor about this. It would be a great opportunity for our church to show that we cared. Our pastor told me that I could have some time to present this to our congregation during the announcement section. On that Sunday, I stood in front of the congregation. I said, "Many of the patients in this nursing home have lived all their lives in this city. Most of their relatives and friends live close by, but they do not visit. You can help feed some of these patients. The staff will tell you which ones need supervision or just some help.

"We as members of this church can show that we care this Thanksgiving. Please sign up for this event. The list is in the narthex. We need only eight volunteers."

When I entered the narthex on Thanksgiving Day, I was surprised and happy to see fourteen names on the list. This made my Thanksgiving. After the Thanksgiving service, we all met in the hall so we could go at the same time, and I explained a little more about what we were going to see and do. Most of them knew where the nursing home was. I asked the few who did not to follow me. I explained to them that this nursing home was one of the few that had an Alzheimer's unit. Anyone on the floor could not just walk away, because all doors had a security lock on them. You had to ask the staff to punch in a code, which opened the door. Anyone coming from the outside had to push a button to get in. This was done to prevent patients from leaving the floor. In addition to this, each patient had a bracelet on his or her arm. If they left the floor, an alarm would go off.

Most of the patients could walk and talk, but all of them needed love and compassion. If someone felt like it, they could hug them, but if they were not sure, they could ask the staff, who would be in the dayroom at the time we got there. For the kitchen staff, this is one of the many assignments they have at the holidays. It is extra work, but they do a good job. I told the volunteers, "If you want, the nursing home offers a free Thanksgiving meal after you have served the residents on the floor." I led the volunteers to the floor. For most of the volunteers, this was their first time in an Alzheimer's unit. It must have been a strange feeling. The volunteers soon began talking with the patients and the staff. The ice was broken. It did not take long before the two large turkeys were brought to the floor. Two church members volunteered to carve them. The staff told them how many slices each patient could have. When the trays came up a little later, I went back to my wife, who ate only pureed food and did not get the turkey meat, and started to feed her. She did not eat much, although I tried. The members of our church seemed to blend in perfectly with the staff and seemed to enjoy this Thanksgiving meal. It gave me a good feeling. When the dinner was over and the tables were cleaned, some of our church members left, while others stayed for a while and chatted with the residents. No one wanted the free meal. I expressed my appreciation to each one of the volunteers and they said that this had been a great experience. I was happy to hear this and stayed with my wife to get her out of her chair for a walk. I am sure that all of our church members will remember this day.

When Christmas approached, I asked our church members again to help out with the Christmas meal. I was not sure if I would get enough people to help out, since Christmas is the biggest holiday of the year. To my surprise, we again got all the volunteers we needed for that day. It gave me a good feeling. This is really what Christmas is all about, caring for others. We did not give presents, but there was no need for that. Our church members gave a part of their happiness to others they had never met before. This was their Christmas gift to the Alzheimer's unit.

I had admitted my wife into this facility with the understanding that she would receive good care, although I knew it never could replace the quality of care she received from me at home. Still, I did not know what kind of care really would be provided in a nursing home. The first four weeks was difficult for the two of us, because my wife was not at home anymore. All the familiar surroundings and routines were gone. Ever since the incident with her bowel movement, I had been on my guard. I knew if this happened once, it would happen again. The reality of nursing-home care took on a different meaning. What about her bladder control? From that day on, my mistrust was established. Christina could not express her need to be cleaned and dried, which included changing underwear and washing the affected areas. She had no one to turn to, because she could not speak. When this all became a bad dream, I knew I had to change, since the nursing home would not. I had to get involved in her care. I also realized that my care was limited to the time I was present at the facility. I could do at least that much and leave the rest up to the nursing home's staff. So I decided to come in earlier and be there when she was still in bed to watch her being washed and dressed and check her just before I left the place. The nurses' aide who usually worked in her section seemed to be friendly.

I came in early that morning while the aides were still on their break. I knew my wife would not mind staying in bed, because she was not an early riser. I kissed her and said good morning, but also checked to make sure she was dry and talked to her. "From now on, I will be here every morning to watch you being washed and dressed. After that, we will walk as we did before and I will check on you before I go home."

The nurses' aide came in and closed the curtains around her. "I have to wash and dress her," she said, indicating to me that I should leave the room.

"I am her husband, and I will stay."

She put a small basket on the nightstand and went to Christina's closet and took out clean clothes. She said to my wife, "I am going to wash you now, starting with your face." Christina did not resist. I remembered when a nurse tried to do this at our home; she would not let her do this. I was happy to see this. It showed that this nurses' aide had the compassion and skills to do this. The aide told me my wife was not eating much and was losing weight. To me, this was not news. She did not eat much at home after she came back from that terrible hospital event. When the aide was done with her face, she removed the nightgown, put a towel over her body, washed her hands and arms, and removed the towel and did her body. Then she rolled her over on her the back, put the towel back on her, and did her legs and feet. When the washing part was done, she started to dress her, bra first, then top, underwear, slacks, knee highs, and shoes. For the dressing part, she had to roll her from left to right and from right to left, several times. I assisted by holding her on her side position. Then she was ready to start the day with me. I thanked the aide and said, "From now on, I will be here every morning."

When we walked out of the room, I knew that this news would travel fast, not only to all the others on the floor but to everyone in the whole building. Since most men did not want to get up early on this unit, we could walk in their section freely and visit with our nursing-home friend, Ed. You could hear Ed every day, "Help me, help me, help me," without interruption. When we stopped in front of him, I introduced my wife to him and I shook his hand. He had white hair, neatly combed, and he was dressed in a white shirt with tie and dark pants. He must have had a good job at one time. As soon as we stopped and spoke with him, he stopped calling for help. He did not make a sound, but we made eye contact. We spent time with Ed every morning, and then we went on our way with the promise we would return the next morning. He kept quiet when we turned around and followed us with his eyes. We did visit Ed every day, until one day he changed his cry for help.

Every afternoon when I came onto the floor, it was always the same confused picture. People all around, male and female patients, gathered in front of the nurses' station. To add to this confusion, Geri chairs were lined up in front of the nurses' station, leaving only a narrow space to move around.

My wife was depressed. She did not eat well. She could not talk to express her needs or the feelings she experienced. She could not tell if she had to go to the bathroom. At home, this was not a problem. I took her to the bathroom. In the nursing home, it was every two hours if they did not forget to do it. She could not ask for orange juice. If she wanted to sit down, she could not locate a chair or ask for one. When I left, she felt alone, and if others tried to talk to her, she could not answer or comprehend the questions.

Every nursing home with an Alzheimer's unit was learning at the cost of the patients. They have changed a little, but not enough. More relatives should visit, not only once a week but regularly, and see and watch their loved ones. Have the courage to look under the blankets and examine the bottoms of their loved ones. Everything was overshadowed by the current problem of toileting. Four times a day was indicated on the schedule for toileting. Three of these interfered with meal time, and the last one was at the changing of the guard. In addition, there was a house rule that no one was allowed to go to the bathroom during meal time. This is wrong. Elderly persons who have trouble with their bladders and bowels can get an urge just from drinking or eating during the early part of a meal.

My wife and I had seen this many times when she was still at home. We were helping other elderly people during a picnic. The intake of food and drink started the process, and it is cruel and dangerous to prevent and stop the body from doing its natural functions. The staff was so used to enforcing this house rule and tried to justify it. One nurses' aide, who was a good and caring person, also wanted to have the last word in a conversation and responded to the statement, "I have to go to the bathroom," by answering, "How can this be? You just took a couple of spoonfuls of food and now you have to go? It does not work that fast. It takes time to go through your system." It was not the current small amount of food. It was this small amount that triggered the ready-to-be-disposed bowel movement.

The new influx of patients who talked back and expressed concerns about this in meetings had results. Changing this rule did not come easily. Finally, the director of nursing made a decision to correct the problem. For each meal, a floater was assigned to help the patients go to the bathroom during mealtime. Was the problem completely corrected? No. A shortage of nursing staff leads to the following excuse: "There is no floater for this meal." So I asked a morning nurses' aide what could be done about keeping my wife dry and clean and indicated that hourly checks would be good enough. She told me that Christina was checked when they came on duty in the morning and if necessary cleaned. Then at breakfast, my wife would be washed and dressed after the break. At lunch she was checked again.

When the aide came in the next morning, she showed me a diaper and said that the charge nurse had decided this was the best way for my wife. I heard about the diaper for adults, but had never seen these items on the drugstore shelf. She showed me how it worked; no more underwear. The thickness of the padding absorbed even a small discharge, but they looked skimpy to me. At home, I had used the very small pads with adhesive on one side to put inside her underwear. I had taken over since she could not do this anymore, and that padding had been heavier than the one on this diaper. It struck me as degrading for an adult to be treated like this. I sensed there should be a better way, the one I used at home.

When Christina entered the nursing home, the medical director had examined her and told me that she was in the most advanced stage of her illness. I felt some pride because I knew I had taken such good care of her at home, longer than any other patient brought to this unit. But it was also scary that the staff did not know how to deal with this advanced stage. At home I had my own bladder—and bowel-control plan, and it worked. I had told the staff this, and they also had it in writing. Their answer was, "We do it our way."

After we washed and dressed her, now with her diaper on, we walked and sat down to rest. I wondered if it felt strange to walk with a piece of plastic between her legs. I wanted to say to that nurse, *Why don't you walk with this kind of diaper between your legs as long as you are on duty on this floor? Then you will know how it feels.* This feeling of frustration and anger stayed with me. But I also knew that I would talk to her and give it a try while I put my best foot forward during that conversation.

"Can I have a moment of your time? I'd like to talk about my wife."

"Certainly. What can I do for you?"

"I have taken care of my wife for many years at home; she is not incontinent. She only needs a little help and guidance, which does not take that much time. I took her to the bathroom every hour. For her bowel movements, she was as steady as clockwork, always in the morning. When she was hospitalized for four days, she was incontinent when she came home, but when she resumed her regular routine at home, the problem was completely gone within a week.

"Could you please try to do that here, also? Every hour, just take her to the bathroom. You already have four toileting times in our schedule. It will be only for the in-between times. She is very advanced in her illness, but she is a quiet person and if guided, she will go to the bathroom."

She listened and replied, "We do not have time to do this."

"It is only for one person. I am not asking you to do this for everyone." But she had made up her mind.

About a year later, the nursing home announced a new program. It was called the bladder control program. One of the routines in this program was that patients who were selected for this were taken to the bathroom every hour. It came too late for my wife.

My wife was very unhappy. She could not talk, but she cried. Her tears spoke more than words could. Before that, the only time I had seen her cry was on our arrival in this country when we were alone in the home that was rented for us by our sponsors. After a very rough boat trip across the Atlantic, our young son, who was only eighteen months old, was so seasick that he had to be taken to the ship's hospital. We changed our plan to travel by train to plane so we could get there quicker and get him better medical care.

When we saw the rented home and the furniture, we had the greatest shock of our lives. If you have never been in this country and the image you have of life in America is the one you have seen in American magazines, it is easy to get the wrong idea. Relatives who came here before you never admitted what a disappointment it was to see the reality of American life. Yes, that was the first time she had cried.

When I saw her cry that afternoon at the nursing home, it brought back that horrible experience. I did know what I had done in the past, but now I just held her in my arms for a very long time.

CHAPTER TEN

Being There for Her

Christina was losing weight and this caught the attention of the staff.

Every day I came in time for dinner to feed her, and I had requested to give her plain yogurt. This was a change for the dietary department, because yogurt was not on their menu list.

It took some time before this new item was approved and purchased and she ate it. I put some extra sugar in it, but it was not really necessary. When the last container was used, it was not reordered; I found this out when a small paper slip was on her tray with the words, "Sorry, the item you order is out of stock." The first time I went to the staff to report this, they called the kitchen, but what could they do? If it was not in stock, they could not send it up. The next time I went to the staff and asked to talk to the supervisor about this matter. When he came in, I explained the situation to him and he said, "I will take care of this." He went to the kitchen and talked to the kitchen supervisor about this said it would be provided the next day. He came back with an eight-ounce container of yogurt that he had purchased from the vending machine. I expressed my appreciation and from that day on, there were no more problems.

I now came into her room in the morning when she was still in bed. I noticed that the two side rails were down. This old hospital bed was much higher from the floor than our bed at home, and this scared me.

At the time of her admission, I had supplied her daily routine to the staff verbally and in writing, and this list included rail protection at night. These high old beds scared me and I went to the charge nurse to express my concern about the fact that the rail was not up. She told me that a study had been done about rails in hospitals and the finding was that the rails up invited more accidents than they prevented. I asked her to get me more details about this report. What percentage was male and what percentage was female? Was their stay in the hospital a long or a short one? Was there any indication about their mental status? She did not know any of these facts about the report and did not want to talk to the doctor about it. I decided to wait until the doctor made his rounds that morning and talk to him about this.

I went back to her room and assisted in dressing my wife. Then we walked up and down the halls waiting for the doctor. When he showed up, I went to him and asked if I could talk to him after his rounds. Fortunately, he did not have many requests that morning. He found us walking in the hall. I explained about the bed rails. He was the only doctor in the nursing home who was an expert in the field of Alzheimer's disease. He agreed with me and went back to the desk to fill out an order to have the two bedrails up when she was in her bed. She never climbed over the rail or fell out of bed in these long years of her stay in the nursing home.

The time between Christmas and New Year's Day is one week, but that time seems to fly. After these weeks, I asked one of the nurses' aides, "If you have off at Christmas, do you also have off on New Year? In other jobs, you have both these holidays off, but what about here?"

She told me that each of the staff had to work on two of the four major holidays. So if you have off at Christmastime, you have to work on New Year's Day. This is also true for the Fourth of July and Thanksgiving. You can put in a request for these days. "I have noticed that this rule does not seem to be applied to all staff," I said. She started to smile and said the nursing office had the final word about the work schedule on these four days. There was another rule about sick days. On the first of January, everyone started with new sick days. Then there were days for emergencies, but you had to bring in written proof of the event.

One day, my wife was ready to leave the room for our walk up and down the halls when suddenly we heard the alarms go off. It scared my wife. The doors slammed shut, making an even more disturbing noise. The nurses' aides came out the rooms in which they were working. The staff from behind the desk joined in to get all the patients back into their rooms.

"What is this?" I asked.

"Oh, it is a drill. You have to bring your wife to her room and stay there." I took my wife to her room. Others were there already and a nurses' aide handed out what looked like army blankets and put one on each bed.

I put my wife on her bed and put my arm around her to make her at ease and told her, "It will be only for a short time. It's only an exercise. I will stay with you until it is over." Our house doctor had told me that she should be shielded from any strong loud noise. This noise was not only loud, but very scary for her condition. A nurse came around to check if all patients were in their rooms. The nurses' aide came and said, "It won't be long; it was a tornado exercise."

There was one resident who knew how to get attention. Besides taking off all her cloths and running naked in the hall, she did not like to walk around with soiled underwear. She took her slacks and underwear off, soiling her hands in the process, sat down on a chair, and cleaned her hands on her top. The staff did not wait too long to clean her. "Is this was the way to get fast action in a nursing home?" I wondered. However, the nurses' aide who first refused to clean my wife must have changed her mind. She overheard me asking another nurses' aide to clean my wife, and she offered to do it.

I was also finding out that quite a few of the staff took advantage of their sick days. When they called in, they were replaced by the staff from other floors, who did not know the routine in this specialized section.

I did not live in the same town as the nursing home. Every day I drove the trip in the morning, and then for the second time in the afternoon. The return trip during the summer was not bad, but in the wintertime with rain and snow, it was difficult. I did not like driving at night. I did not mind driving in snow, but icy roads with freezing rain kept me at home against my will. Usually when the road conditions were bad, there were not too many drivers on the highways. There was a new kind of car with four-wheel drive. Most of the drivers of these new cars drove on snow and icy roads as if it was summertime. It scared me to see these cars passing on the roads with icy conditions. If I was hit by one of these cars, not only would I lose my transportation but also I could be hurt. The weather channel was constantly providing road conditions and so was the radio, but each had different amounts of snow forecast. Each person you talked to had different weather stories, so you did not know what to believe and had to use your own judgment.

When this happened the first time, I called my pastor and he offered to take me to the nursing home and pick me up later. He was a caring person and showed that by his actions. Snow, I could handle, as long as it was not in excess of three or four inches. We had lived in states where three months of snow was normal, but they had all the equipment to take care of the snowfall. When it snowed, I came in to visit, while some of the staff called out and stayed home. The only time I stayed home was when the snow was drifting in the street. Our driveway was so filled with snow that no matter what you did, you could not get out even if you cleaned the driveway because of the snowdrifts in the street.

I came into Christina's room one morning and she was the only one left in bed. I went on with our normal routine. I kissed her and told her about cleaning the driveway the night before and then the snow plough came and I had to clean the entrance again. She had helped me in the past, but not since she had Alzheimer's disease. I checked to see if she was dry, and went to her closet and chest of drawers to take out her clothes for that day. While I waited, I talked some more until the nurses' aide came. Then I talked to her about the snow again.

As a general rule, the nurses' aides on this floor were caring persons. A few knew about Alzheimer's disease from experience in their own family, which made a great difference. When the aide came in, she saw that I had already put out my wife's clothes for the day. The rest she would do. After washing her face, hands, and arms, she did her body. I noticed a discoloration of Christina's skin on the lower part of her body and upper insides of both her thighs. "What is this and how did it get there?" I asked.

"That is diaper rash," she said.

"Diaper rash? I associate that with babies."

"Yes, but it is quite common for incontinent elderly."

I thought about how we had had three children and how I had helped to change our firstborn. Christina took the soiled diaper off and I rinsed it out in a pail of water. At that time, we did not have disposable diapers. But none of our three children had ever had diaper rash. "What are you going to do about this?" I asked.

"Oh, I put some baby powder on it, and it should be gone by tomorrow." Tomorrow came, but the rash was still there.

"What will be the next treatment to take care of this?"

"I will put some A&D ointment on it."

The next day there was no improvement, and the day after that, there was another nurses' aide who rolled my wife over so that I could see her buttocks. I looked and saw the start of an open sore. Right away, memories came back from the short stay in the hospital. I became upset and angry but remembered that the hospital nurse had said zinc oxide cream would take care of it, and it really did.

"What can we do now about this open sore?" I asked.

"We can only put A&D on it for now. I have to talk to the doctor about this."

After Christina was dressed, I tried to conceal my anger and went to the charge nurse and explained the situation and requested a meeting with the supervisor; the charge nurse knew very well that I was angry. She called me later while I was walking with my wife in the halls and told me that the meeting was set for 9:00 a.m. the next morning.

In the small meeting room were three staff members, the supervisor, the charge nurse, and the social worker. When I saw this group, my mind flashed, there were three of them and only me? They also knew that I was angry about my wife's treatment. I tried to control myself and started to explain again what had happened in the last three days and my experience in the short stay at the hospital before she came to the nursing home. In addition, I mentioned the poor quality of the lining in the diapers currently used and how I handled my wife's bladder and bowel control at home.

"I would like to propose to you that the problem of the diapers can be easily solved by me without any cost to the nursing home. I will provide a diaper with a heavier absorption. I have found a brand that will do the job." I asked their permission to bring in a box containing about a hundred good diapers. The next point was the cream, for which I referred to the visiting hospital nurse. This cream had healed her pretty fast when she had open sores after her hospital visit. Each of them tried to defend or make excuses for what had happened, but the supervisor made the final decision to let me bring in the diapers. He would talk to the doctor about the cream to be applied to the open sore. I expressed my appreciation to the group. I went to the medical supply and equipment store to get the first box of diapers. After I had used four boxes, the nursing home did not use the poor quality diapers anymore but used good ones like I had.

The doctor had done more than I asked for. On the order, he had prescribed not only the cream to be applied at every shift but also a lamb's fleece to sit on in her chair. Little did I know that the fleece was such a hot item in the Alzheimer's unit.

The unit is known not only for its confused atmosphere, but also for the fact that patients take items from other patients and bring them to different rooms, in which they wander or bring things into their own rooms and forget about them.

When Christina was not walking, she was usually sitting in her room or out in the hall where I could watch her most of the time. The tray was in a down position so no one could use it. The fleece was always gone when I came in the morning or in the afternoon. The staff always had a good idea of who had taken it or where to find it, and I retraced it myself more than once. Lamb's fleece seems to have a great appeal. I used it to cover our car's front seat. It is cool in the summer, and in the winter you never feel a cold seat. It minimizes the pressure between buttocks and the seat of a chair. The day came that no one could find it. The fleece was gone.

Did the patients outsmart us? To replace the lamb's fleece with an egg-crate cushion with a cover was the next best thing. As soon as I had it, I put my wife's initials on the back of the label so there could not be any argument about the ownership.

One afternoon I found Christina sitting in the wrong chair. I knew she could not have done this. Most likely at the changing of the guard at 3:00 p.m., they took the first chair available and put her in it. There was no cushion on the chair. I looked in a couple of rooms and saw it. Now I had to get the cushion under her, but how? I could not do this alone. I needed help, and every staff member was at the orientation meeting.

You have to take time to change an Alzheimer's patient from a sitting position to a standing one. Most of us do this without thinking about it, but this was not the case for my wife in her advanced condition. I needed another person to help me. There was no staff member in sight, but there was a nurse, whom I will call Sherry, who was visiting her mother after she had finished her work at a local nearby hospital. I had talked to her before. We knew each other and knew about this terrible disease. In addition to her mother, Sherry had an aunt on the Alzheimer's floor. My wife was crying and upset. I put my arm around her and with the other I motioned to Sherry. I asked her to hold my wife on one side while I held her on the other. We lifted her from the chair, moved her over to the right chair, put the cushion on the seat, and let her down.

When we did this, we noticed the odor. I told her that after the shift change, they did not really pay too much attention if a patient needed to be cleaned. The shift that was leaving left the job for the next shift. The new shift believed the last shift should have taken care of it. My wife had been sitting in her bowel movement for how long? We found a caring nurses' aide who took care of my wife and cleaned her.

Sherry had told me that she had put her mother in a first-class nursing home that had an Alzheimer's research department. It sounded impressive and she said that the quality of care was much better in that nursing home, but after her mother had spent all her savings she was transferred to this nursing home. I knew what she meant by "spending down." Each state now has laws in place resulting from the Omnibus Reconciliation Act, which was approved by Congress. If you needed to place your spouse in a nursing home because you could not take care of her anymore and the doctor had told you that this was the only way she could be taken care of, the next step was to find one. Then a contract stating the rights and obligations of both parties should be drawn up and signed. Nursing homes have waiting lists that are not expressed in weeks or months, but years. If you have savings accumulated during the years you worked and intended to use these savings to enjoy your retirement, you are wrong. The Republican Congress came up with a "contract" not intended to help citizens, but to benefit the nursing-home industry so they could do what they wanted, as well as the health insurance companies. The Republican Congress' plan stated that in order for individuals in long-term care to qualify for medical assistance, they first had to spend a significant part of their savings and assets. This was referred to as "spending down." This meant you could get a loved one into a nursing home ahead of the waiting list by paying the cost for the nursing home from your savings or turning over your assets. Once in the nursing home, you had to submit a formal statement, documented with financial statements, listing all your combined assets and submit it to the Public Welfare Department of your state, which would determine your total countable, documented net resources. The Omnibus Reconciliation Act determined which part should be protected for the spouse remaining at home. This was subject to a maximum. In other words if you had more resources than the maximum, they were not protected. Is it right to single out one illness and treat it totally differently from any other illness? No. Spending down is a violation of human rights, as stated in Article 25 of the Universal Declaration of Human Rights, which was signed by our country, the United States of America. It asserts that everyone has the right to a standard of living adequate for the health and well-being of himself and of his family, including food, clothing, housing, medical care, and necessary social services, as well as the right to security in the event of unemployment, sickness, widowhood, old age, or other lack of livelihood in circumstances beyond a person's control. The Universal Declaration of Human Rights is about rights. In America, we have about thirty million Americans who do not have any health insurance. This means that our senators and representatives, both federal and state, are violators of our human rights.

One morning many years ago, Christina woke with a pain in her ear. I cleaned it, but it did not solve the problem. I did not know what to do. Our doctor did not have the equipment to clean her ear. Going to the emergency room did not enter my mind. Our pastor had given me the name of a specialist in that field and recommended him in case she might need him. The pain did not go away, so I called this doctor early in the morning and explained our situation to him. His response was so warm and gentle that I will never forget it. Normally he did not work on Saturdays, but he agreed to meet us at 9:00 a.m. in his office.

We were there before he was and waited in our car and followed him into his office, where I had to fill out forms. At that time, Christina could still follow simple instructions, and the otolaryngologist was quite familiar with Alzheimer's disease, which was unusual. It was a blessing for us. He put her in a chair and talked to her. I was always in front of her so she could see me. He started the vacuum at a distance so that the noise would not be that intense for her and came slowly closer to get her used it. She was scared and I offered to stand at her side and hold her hand to give her security. The doctor succeeded in vacuuming all the wax out and gave her medication. That was then, but now we had not only ear problems, but also bladder and bowel trouble, in a very different and uncomfortable situation.

Chapter Eleven

Holding On

Our son came for a visit and offered me a break. He would visit his mother as I did in the morning and afternoon. I stayed home for two days. I appreciated this very much. The staff worked a regular shift, with days off and holidays off. I worked every day, including Saturday, Sunday, and holidays. It was a lot of travel time. Many visitors saw me every time they came. Someone made the remark, "You must live close by." When I told them how many miles I traveled each day to visit my wife, there was no reply. I traveled about twenty thousand miles a year to see her each day.

After my son left, I resumed the daily routine. When we took a rest and sat down on her bed, she suddenly said, "Where is Olof?" Her words were so distinct. I was not just surprised; I was flabbergasted. I smiled at her. She had not spoken a word in a long time, and now these three words? It had happened before. The ability to speak returns only for a short time. I took her hands and told her that he had come to visit her and now had gone back to work. There was silence. Then tears came to my eyes. I pulled her toward me and held her for quite some time. When our son returned about four weeks later and took care of her again, there was no reaction, no words—just silence.

We were resting in the hall after our walk, and a priest passed. He came every morning to visit and to bless certain patients. He was over eighty years old, and this was now part of his job. Suddenly my wife looked at him and started to laugh. He stopped and looked at her. Not knowing how to react, he responded with, "God bless you."

I thanked him, and after that day whenever I saw him I said, "Good morning, Father."

I came in one day and found Christina sleeping in her chair. I asked the staff, "Did she walk already?" "No," was the answer. I pulled up a chair and put it next to her. I did not wake her up. The staff would do this. I once read a book written by a person about his early experience with Alzheimer's disease. He wrote, "It is a terrible feeling to wake up. You can't compare it with a normal wake-up. You are lost; everything seems strange. You don't know which direction you have to go. You are frightened. It feels like you are in complete darkness. It takes time to adjust."

I let her sleep until she opened her eyes and looked around and saw me. I put my hand on her hand. Then I saw that her cushion was not on the seat, but at the back of the chair. The only way to solve this was to take her out the chair and start walking. It was morning, so we could walk on the other side while the men were still in bed. For some reason she did not like to walk this morning, and when we returned, the chair was gone. We went to her room and there it was, but no cushion. We found a nurses' aide in her section and asked, "Do you know where her cushion is?"

"Yes. Sarah's daughter used the chair and might have left the cushion in her room. Let me go and check it." She came back with the cushion and I thanked her for finding it.

We had an encounter with a wild madman. All men were told, "Do not go into the ladies' section," but they still did it. Some found a bed and rested on it, and if the women came in, it was trouble. The patients knew to get a staff member to get a man out their bed and tell him to return to his own section. For some reason, this man could not get out of his wheelchair. I saw him coming from his section, passing the nurses' station, and going in our direction—toward my wife. He was very strong and used his arms and hands as weapons to lash out at patients in his path of travel. He was in an angry mood.

Danny, the male charge nurse, was giving out medications to the patients at that time but always kept an eye on the man, who was a dangerous troublemaker. I ran to Danny and told him that our "friend" Henry was on his way to my wife and seemed to be in a bad mood. We ran back together and Danny pulled him backward while he was trying to move on toward his objective. It was a blessing that Danny was much stronger than Henry and had some way to get him out of situations where he might hurt patients or break bones. He pulled Henry all the way back to his room while he was trying to go forward. Danny put him in his room and went to the medicine cart and gave him an injection. It calmed him down pretty fast. One ounce of prevention is better than a pound of cure. I could only hope that Danny would be here if Henry acted out when I was not here to look after my wife.

When the food trays came, the nursing home got quiet. The patients who can eat without help were busy satisfying their appetite. Others who did not like what was on their plates used this opportunity to make trouble and take their disappointment over the menu out on others by making insulting remarks or disturbing the peaceful atmosphere. They pushed their plates across the table where somebody else was enjoying the meal or spilled a glass of juice over the table. The nurses' aide, who was feeding a few patients, one on the left and one on the right of her, could control the troublemakers. Others who were not able to feed themselves were put in very small groups along the wall, in view of the nurses' station. My wife was in the last group. I put the tray on the table and took one plate or container at a time. She ate slowly, as she always had done, peacefully and contentedly. She enjoyed her food. She was not put on a special diet. The menu for the whole week was posted on the bulletin board, but most patients did not pay attention to it. Some of them had lost the ability to read and comprehend what was printed.

On weekdays, the food was fair, but on Saturdays and Sundays, it was terrible. After the first weekend, I was well prepared for the next; I brought extra food to replace the items that were no good. There was one mystery item. It looked like soft dough and had a strange color. On the plate, it leveled out like a pancake and looked like Elmer's glue. I never tasted it. It looked disgusting. I tasted the other food on her tray before I offered it to her. As a general rule, the food tasted good on the weekdays. I also supplemented her diet with cookies and fruit juice from home. When she did not want to eat anymore, I brought the tray to the staff and went back to her, and we walked.

We came upon a woman who told me we had met before and my wife did not swear and I was a nice man. Her name was Martha. She was ninety-six years old, could walk and talk and eat by herself, and did not have Alzheimer's. Yet she was on the Alzheimer's unit. When we walked up and down the halls, we sometimes saw her in her room. When I knocked at the door, she would invite us in for a visit. She was very amicable and social. It made a nice change to see her and communicate with her. One day while we were talking she said to me, "I'd like to see your home. It must be spick and span." I suppose she made that assumption because Christina's room was always tidy.

Chapter Twelve

Falls and Breaks

I can still remember that Saturday afternoon when I entered the floor of the Alzheimer's unit. Danny was waiting for me and told me that about twenty minutes before, my wife had fallen and had broken her hip. We walked to her room and there she was in very great pain. I looked at her and carefully took her hand and talked to her. Then I turned to the Danny and said, "How could this happen? She was supposed to be resting in a chair. The first shift should have made sure she was secure. If they did not do it, you should have done it. I know you come in early and should have noticed this. You know how hectic it is at that time on Saturday."

He ignored the remark and said, "Henry had another one of his outbursts. Your wife was just walking there when it happened. He pushed her and she fell, which resulted in a hip fracture." The fear I had had for some time had now become a reality. This accident was due to neglect on the part of the nursing-home staff on both shifts. I knew that they left early on weekends, but their hurry to get out resulted in an unnecessary accident. I was sure she was not the only one this wild man had knocked down. I just knew more than the casual visitor because I came there every day. The staff would only say, "Oh she fell and broke her hip." If they had put her in a chair and waited until the new shift was ready to take control, my wife would not have broken her hip. I know sometimes they fall on their own account as a result of their illness. My wife did that at home, too, but did not break her hip. The Alzheimer's units have a higher-than-average rate of accidents, but with more staff, this could certainly be reduced. The Alzheimer's unit has a little bit more staff than other floors, but still not enough to prevent unnecessary accidents and remove patients with violent behavior pattern from the area.

The ambulance attendants came into the room and transferred her from the bed to the stretcher. She was in more pain during this move. She went to a downtown hospital and I followed in my car. It had started to rain by the buckets. I looked for a place to park. One car had taken two spaces and there were no spaces left. So I parked my car behind two other cars and left my blinkers on. When I walked into the emergency room, I saw stretchers, but not my wife. I went to the emergency desk. There were four persons in front of me asking questions. I looked around and saw a small office with only one person in it and no one else. I wanted to call our children and found a pay phone, but I did not have my reading glasses. Then I changed my mind. Our pastor had told me, "If you ever have to go to a hospital again, call me." This was after our first experience in the hospital. I left the pay phone and went to the small, quiet office, knocked at the door, and told the person in the office that I needed to call our pastor but I did not remember his phone number. My wife had been taken somewhere in the hospital, but I didn't know where.

She agreed to let me use the phone if I kept the call short. I told her our pastor's name and that he had served as a chaplain in this hospital. She found the number and dialed it for me.

In spite of all the pressure, shock, and confusion, this was a quiet place surrounded by a lot of pain and misery. A caring and compassionate hospital employee was helping me. It gave me a good feeling. From this point, I still could see the rain coming down and could keep an eye on my car in case anybody needed me to move it.

"Thank you very much. I really appreciate what you did."

"You are welcome."

I told our pastor what had happened at the nursing home. He told me that he was on his way to a meeting but would call the chaplaincy office and would ask somebody to see me. After I hung up and expressed my appreciation again to the woman, I suddenly saw a car moving out, leaving a spot for me to pull in. I ran out, parked our car, and ran back. It was still pouring. The emergency overhang gave me little protection from the rain.

When I came back in, I saw a sister looking around and asking questions. "Are you looking for me?"

"My name is Sister Martha. I will bring you to your wife."

We left the emergency room and walked into a holding room. There, she was crying and in severe pain. All that I could do at that moment was to let her feel that I was there for her. She could not talk, but she sensed that I was with her. The sister felt Christina's forehead, and then took a paper towel, held it under the cold faucet, and put in on her forehead. Then she left and came back with a doctor to give my wife an injection. I saw the needle going in pretty deep. After fifteen minutes, Christina stopped crying and fell asleep. Then she was taken to the X-ray room. I waited in the waiting room, watching staff come and go. When she returned, blood samples were taken and she was given an EKG. After that, she was transferred to the seventh floor.

I asked, "When will the surgery be?" I was told it could be two or three hours. So I waited. After midnight, a nurse came and told me, "Why don't you go home and call us at 7:00 a.m. tomorrow morning?" When I left, it was not raining anymore. The downtown streets were deserted. This was the first time that I had driven our car without seeing any other cars.

I called early on Sunday morning and was told the surgery would be between 11:30 and noon. I decided to go to the hospital and keep Christina company. She was moving her right leg in an unusual motion. The left leg was in traction, which caused her pain. The nurse told me that she had just received a pain injection. All I could do was hold her hands and talk to her.

Our pastor called and said he would be over after the service. When he arrived, I was so emotional that I cried. He put his arms around me. He also kept my wife's right leg from moving and got a swab to clean her palate and mouth. Then he went to the nurses' station and asked for another shot of painkiller, which she received almost immediately. It pays to have a pastor who had volunteered as a chaplain. My wife was in the first bed but there was another one occupied by an elderly woman whose daughter was visiting and talking loudly. It sounded like they were having an argument about care and money. The daughter said, "You do not know what happened to you; they found you unconscious in your house." The mother replied, "You are trying to control me." This went on and on. They were so loud that I asked them to lower their voices because my wife was in severe pain and needed rest and sleep. After the daughter left, a couple in red scarves came in and stayed for a short time. Then their pastor came. The last visitor was a young girl who talked about her boyfriend, whom she met a few months before. They were going to get married, and she asked Grandma to pay for the wedding. Fortunately my wife slept through this whole event.

An orderly came into the room and told me that he had to take my wife to the operating room. In order to do this, he had to unplug the cord of the electrical bed. For some reason, he had a lot of trouble doing this. The plastic bottle fell off the hook and onto the bed. I left the room until he had all things under control and came out of the room with the bed. It was past 4:00 p.m. when he took her down to prepare her for surgery. The nurse told me to report to a waiting room and wait for a call. After getting lost and having to ask for directions, I found the spot. Three other families were already there. When the phone rang, I picked it up and was told that all further information about the surgery would be directed to this extension.

I went outside and noticed two other waiting rooms. One was for the bypass surgery. The other did not have any indication about its use; each one of these two rooms had much better furniture. Could it be that the unmarked one was for patients who would go to private rooms? As time went by, the other families left and I was alone, so I could not leave the room anymore in case the phone rang. It was 5:45 p.m. when I got a call that the surgery had started.

How long I waited I do not remember, but finally the phone rang and I was told the surgeon was coming down to see me. He told me that Christina had had a spinal injection and was talking the whole time. I did not understand what he meant by "talking" since Christina could not talk. I had had surgery with a spinal injection, but I was out cold. He told me she would walk again. The ball socket had snapped off, but was replaced with a steel one, and a rod was inserted into the hipbone.

"How large was the incision?"

"About ten inches."

"How did you know the exact size of the socket to be replaced?"

"By carefully measuring it."

She had to stay in bed for about six weeks and would stay in the recovery room now. "Why don't you get something to eat?" he advised.

"Will you write a prescription for cream for the sore spots on her buttocks and instruct the nurses to keep her dry and clean?"

"Yes, I will."

"Thank you very much, Doctor."

This was the first time I had been in the hospital cafeteria. It was not busy and I had plenty of time to look at the available dishes. I took my time and made a selection. I found a good spot to sit where I could overlook the whole cafeteria. I started to eat. Then I saw our pastor walking in. He looked at my plate and said, "I will try some of that, too." He came and sat with me. I told him how long we had had to wait before my wife was taken into surgery. "It reminds me of triage, an uncommon word that is used in field hospitals and practiced in emergency rooms all over our country. It is a process that sorts patients and treats them according to need, so that those with the highest possibility of surviving are helped first."

"The staff kept her 'on hold' for the remainder of Saturday and about sixteen hours on Sunday. She suffered longer than the others, who were helped first," I said.

"Just look at the emergency rooms. They are overloaded and understaffed, but no one in the medical field is going to change it. After medical school, the doctors have to do their residency. This term dates back to the time when they really lived in the hospital, but that was over a hundred years ago."

"We live in the past," I said. Look at other countries:

- Australia limits their residency doctors to seventy-five hours a week.
- The European Union designated a maximum forty-eight hour week in 2003.
- The United Kingdom has a fifty-six-hour weekly limit.
- Denmark has a forty-five hour weekly limit.

The United States does not even work to achieve a nationwide solution. The bottom line, as usual in our country, is money. Where could the hospital industry get any cheaper labor than by working their doctors to a point where the health of a patient is at risk? A study has proven that resident doctors who work twenty-four hours in a row have a cognitive performance of a person who has a blood alcohol level of 0.10. The legal limit in most states is 0.08, so these doctors are performing like people legally under the influence. Another study reported that forty percent of mistakes were due to fatigue, and thirty percent of the resident doctors who reported mistakes said that their errors had resulted in the death of a patient. The uninsured health-care citizens, about thirty million, depend on emergency room services for health care. This accounts for about thirty percent of the patients in this hospital. In the United States, the number of elderly has greatly increased and this group usually more than one complaint, which takes more time to check. Many patients are sicker than in the past. This is also true for patients admitted to nursing homes. Other reasons for poor hospital care are: A shortage of beds, a shortage of nurses, and a shortage of hospitals. Many hospitals have closed in the last twenty years. As a result, more primary care and family physicians are sending patients for urgent care to emergency rooms.

We talk and write about health-care problems, but then it stops and there is no action to improve it. Before too long, another unspoken or publicly mentioned danger will be the shortage of medical doctors. Who wants to study and do their internships under the existing conditions, pay off the medical school loans and become employees of the health-care industry? The price is paid by the patients. At least sixty thousand die needlessly each year in emergency rooms and hospitals due to the flaws in our medical/health-care system.

We talked some more and when we were done eating, the pastor suggested we go upstairs and ask the nurses at what time my wife would come back. When we went upstairs and I looked into her room, the bed was empty. We went to the nurses' station and asked at what time she would be coming up. The nurse had no information, but called the recovery room and found out that she was on her way up. Christina's room was close to the nurses' station, and soon we saw her coming out of the elevator. It took a little while to get her settled in the room. When we came in, she was not awake. Our pastor suggested to me, "You better go home and return tomorrow."

When I arrived the next day, I checked with the nurses' station and was told Christina had a 101-degree fever. I went into her room and found a wet washcloth on her forehead; it was not cold anymore, so I removed it. I put it under the cold water faucet let it run and squeezed it so that it would not drip but still be cool enough to do the job of lowering the fever. She did not move at all. I took a chair, put it next to her bed, and held her hand. Around five o'clock, her tray came up and was put in front of her on an adjustable table. It looked good. There was a nice plate and a good quality knife, fork, and spoon with a linen napkin. The food looked appetizing: small baked potatoes, vegetables, good-smelling meat. It was quite different from the nursing home, almost like day and night. There was one thing wrong though; it was not pureed. She could not eat it this way. I called the nurse and told her about it. She took it away and said, "Oh, no. We will have another one in about forty minutes. About an hour later, there was no tray, and I called again. I was told it had to be changed in the computer. At 7:00 p.m., still no tray, so I asked the nurse to give me the name and extension of the kitchen supervisor. No one knew the name or extension. I went to the charge nurse and was really upset and let her have it and asked for the director of nursing to come and see me. Another hour passed.

When the director of nursing arrived, she knew what this was all about and started to explain that this was the first day of a nurse who had just passed her RN exam and had started a new job working on this shift. This made sense. I had seen and talked to her. She took good care of my wife and was compassionate. She kept her clean and dry and put the cream on as I had requested. Every time the staff had requested a new tray, it had come up, but it was not pureed. Instead of delivering it, it was left at the nurses' station. The new nurse was not told that if a menu had to be changed, it had to be done by changing the patient's data in the computer. The director of nursing told me that she would change my wife's menu in the computer. After we finished talking, it was past 9:00 p.m. We looked at Christina. She was sound asleep and we decided to let her sleep.

The next morning, although it was not visiting time, I was back at the hospital, because I had called the surgeon's office and was told he would be in the hospital at 8:00 a.m. I told the receptionist that Dr. Smith would be in the hospital according to his office staff. She said, "Let me check the list of all the doctors who are in the hospital." His name was not on the list. She called him over the intercom—no reply. She waited and called for a second time but got no response. I gave my wife's name and room number and said I would be in her room. My wife was awake and did not show any sign of pain or discomfort. She had a piece of sturdy foam between her legs. The outside had a curvature to hold her legs in place and four straps to keep her legs attached to the foam.

I held her hands and talked to her. Before I knew it; it was lunch time. The nurses took her out of the bed and put her in a chair so I could feed her. I watched her face and she did not show any sign of pain during the transfer. I was happy about this. When she had finished her meal, the tray was removed and she was put back in bed. The nurses washed her bottom and put the cream on. I expressed my appreciation to the two nurses.

At home, I had a quick lunch and drove back to the hospital. When I came to the floor, I saw that the new shift was already on duty. I looked for the charge nurse from yesterday. I apologized for my behavior. She replied, "That's okay; I have been there. I know what it's like."

The doctor called and told me that for the next two days, Christina would be evaluated by the physical therapy department. This was not news to me, because I had seen my wife's name on the list. I asked him if it was possible to keep her a few days longer to get more therapy, because the care was so much better than in the nursing home. "It will come out your own pocket."

"I will gladly pay those extra days and would appreciate it if you would do this for her and me."

As I was getting ready to go to the hospital the next afternoon, I got a call from the nursing home and was told, "Your wife is here in the nursing home. She is in her bed."

"How is this possible? The doctor had told me that today she would be evaluated by the physical therapy department of the hospital." No reply.

"Medicaid will pay for the surgery and hospitalization because it was an accident with injury."

I was deeply disappointed in the surgeon and the physical therapy department of the hospital. It was not the first time that I found out that medical technicians were confused when they had to deal with an Alzheimer's patient. Physical therapists' routine of giving instructions and asking questions to get patients' reactions is a necessary part of their job. When this established routine is suddenly gone, what can they do? After this phone call, I drove to the nursing home and was met by a staff LPN who told me that my wife had to stay in bed for six weeks. This frightened me. I was not concerned about the medication because the nursing home had to follow the doctor's instructions. I knew when I saw her in pain I could ask for pain medication and they had to give it to her. But what about pressure sores?

When I came into her room she was awake and I kissed her, held her hand, and talked to her. The foam between her legs was still there. I found out that she only had an underpad on, so I could easily check if she was dry and not soiled. I had a radio/tape player locked in her nightstand. I kept it locked up because if some of the patients saw it they would move it to another place. I put the tape in. It was light classical music. When she heard the music, she started to move her arms like a conductor of an orchestra. I was flabbergasted. She used to do this at home too when she was in a happy mood.

Then a nurses' assistant came in and was going to give Christina her bath. I made a remark about the flimsy quality of her underpad. She said she would get a better one. She put the cream on. Later that morning, Christina had a bowel movement, so I looked for the nurses' assistant and found her. She cleaned her up while I held her in the side position.

Christina got other medication than for pain. When the LPN came in with the medication, I asked her to crush the pill and then put it in applesauce or any baby food she had was on her medicine cart.

The regular charge nurse told me that the nursing-home physical therapy department would evaluate Christina. The next morning before visiting my wife, I went to the physical therapy department and waited outside the office. I could see not only the tiny administrative office but also the very small therapy room. It looked as if this area had been designed to be offices, not a therapy room. One wall must have been removed to make it larger. The nursing home had not been built with a physical therapy department. Nursing homes should be designed to the needs of their patients and not be just copies of hospitals with some modifications. For patients who have broken a hip and needed to exercise to walk again, this was not the right place. There was a device with two parallel bars, but this could not be used for my wife in her advanced condition of Alzheimer's. When it was my turn to see the therapist, I told her about my wife and that I visited her twice a day. Right from the start, there seemed to be chemistry between the therapist and me. We talked openly about my wife's condition. She told me that the main part of her therapy would be on Christina's floor twice a day. She would have one session during the seven-to-three shift and the other on the three-to-eleven shift. Once a week, Christina would be brought down here to evaluate her progress. The physical therapist also said that Christina was recovering pretty well from her surgery. I agreed with the schedule because the halls on the women's wing were almost deserted in the morning. She also told me that Christina would be using a walker with two supports. After our talk, I went to Christina's room and told her that she was going to walk today; I waited until the nursing assistant came to wash and dress her. After that was taken care of, two restorative assistants came and supported her on the left and right and moved her slowly over to the edge of the bed so that her feet were on the floor. They pulled her up to get her in a standing position. With the help of the two, she stood on her own for the first time since she'd been injured by the accident. To get her hands on each side of the walker was not so easy. It took some time to get it across to her. This was all new to her. With support from the left and the right, she walked from her bed to the door, waited there, and was turned around slowly and walked back to her bed. This was a distance of eighteen feet. I was impressed and told her, "You are doing well."

On Saturdays and Sundays there were no restorative assistants available. The physical therapy department, the nursing-home administrator, the director and the assistant director of nursing, and the charges nurses of the seven-to-three shift were off. The maintenance department had only one person for the first and second shift.

The next week, Christina walked better and increased the distance she walked up to one hundred feet, but she did not get any exercise in the afternoon. One of the many problems with Alzheimer's patients is that they cannot learn new things, but she did prove that she could walk. People who do not have Alzheimer's and are in the same age group have difficulty regaining the ability to walk, but repetition day-in, day-out will bring them back to normal walking ability. My wife had basically the same problems. She did not walk close enough to the front bar of the walker. It looked as if she was pushing it, but the restorative assistants were holding her.

I was always in front of her, walking backward to encourage her to come along. With the up and downs in her progress, she walked up to three hundred feet. Had they given her practice in the afternoon, it would have made a big difference.

The weekly visits to the physical therapy department were different. I did not understand why she had to go there. If the staff wanted to see her progress, all they had to do was come upstairs and watch her, not only once but at different times. This would have been a better evaluation. They might have noticed the difference and could have raised the question as to why the afternoon exercise was omitted. There was also a great difference in environment. Her floor was almost empty on the women's side. Downstairs in the physical therapy department, it was too crowded and definitely created fear in my wife's mind that somebody might hurt her again, making her reluctant to move. When I asked the question more than once, "Why does she not walk in the afternoon as recommended by the physical therapy department?" I was told over and over, "We do not have the time."

What made me so angry was that the charge nurse accepted this and did not take any action to correct it. I was there long enough in the afternoon that I could help. This was a fatal mistake; patients recovering from broken hip need a lot of exercises to restore their walking ability, but this shift got away with it. In other places of employment, when you tell your boss, "I do not have time to do that job," you will be told, "Well, then, you make time. If you don't do it, out you go." In the nursing-home industry, the nurses can get away with it.

I was disappointed but not surprised when the physical therapist told me, "Your wife will be discharged from maintenance therapy by the end of this month. We know that your wife is doing well with the restorative assistants on her floor. Unfortunately, she is not ambulating that well in our therapy department for whatever reason. It could be environmental or the time of day. It is counterproductive to continue unsuccessful attempts or reinforce poor techniques. The physical therapy will continue on her floor.

"It has been a pleasure working with you and your wife. I wish there was more I could do for your wife, but there is nothing at the present time. I respect the commitment you have made to ensure that your wife does not lose ground. I wish the best for both of you."

Christina continued walking in the mornings. If she walked in the afternoon, it was only three or four times. *So much for following recommendations from the therapy department in a nursing home,* I thought.

One morning, while I was watching the morning news at home, the telephone rang. It was the charge nurse with a very short message. "Your wife is not doing so well." I had heard that such a short message was very serious; most of the time it was a euphemistic way of telling you that she was in a very critical or a life-threatening condition. While I was driving, all kinds of terrible ideas came to my mind. *Could it be that this was the last time I would see her alive? Was this another transient ischemic attack?* She had had these before when I took care of her at home. I reported this to our family doctor who told me that it was a transient ischemic attack, or TIA, a term I had never heard before. My wife had the habit of taking one aspirin a day for many years and said an ounce of prevention is better than a pound of cure. I had continued to do that for her, but I had to crush up the pill. Now all I could wonder was, *Was this a stroke or a heart attack?* The early morning traffic was very heavy. It was slow due to all the school bus traffic. Our area was a nice area with homes that were still affordable. The school systems were good, and it was a good place to raise a family. When I entered her room I could not see her bed. It was surrounded by many people dressed in white coats. I was told what had happened. She was walking in the hall and suddenly started to shake and tremble and fell down. They had put an oxygen mask on her. The doctor did not tell me his diagnosis, but told me that an ambulance was on its way to take her to the new medical center where the latest magnetic resonance imaging machine would take pictures of her head. The ambulance crew transferred her to the litter. I asked if I could follow them, because I did not know where this new medical center was located. The charge nurse told me on my way out that this MRI was the best and the latest in this area. We drove through the center of town, then on a new divided highway which took us out the city to the new medical center. It was quite impressive to see all the buildings, including the beautifully designed MRI building, which had its own entrance and parking facilities. I was right behind the ambulance and made it in time to follow the litter into the building. The halls were three times as wide as in the nursing home, with a carpeted floor and large windows. If felt more like a corporate headquarters building than a hospital. In the waiting room, which was also very large and quite different from waiting rooms in other health facilities, the ambulance crew gave the envelope with instructions to the staff, which took over from that point. We did not have to wait. I was surprised. *What service. Was I dreaming or was this for real?* I explained to the staff that Christina was in the advanced stages of Alzheimer's and had lost, as a result of this illness, her ability to follow instructions. I asked if I could stay with her as long as possible. There were no objections.

We went into the MRI room. This was the first time I had ever seen this type of machine. I had only seen pictures of it. She was put on the track. Her head was supported so it could not move, but here was a problem. If she was frightened for some reason in this small tube, she would move her head and the image would not be good. I left the room and went with the technician to his room where I could see the cross sections of her head, but she moved her head. The track was stopped. The supports for her head were adjusted. We started all over. I saw the pictures of her head until the job was done. The images were taken to the specialist. We had to wait for his diagnosis. When the doctor came in, he told me that there was no sign of bleeding in the brain, explaining that there are two kinds of strokes. In one case, the blood vessel ruptures and that is called a hemorrhagic stroke. The other is a trombonist stroke, when a blood clot blocks a cerebral artery. Now I knew at least what this was all about and expressed my appreciation to the doctor and the staff. The ambulance took her back to the nursing home and I drove.

When I got back to the nursing home, I was told that during the fall, Christina had sprained her ankle and had to stay in bed. She would receive whirlpool treatments. Two weeks of not being able to exercise would be bad for her. She would be kept in bed. This would affect her recovery. I was very depressed to hear of this. What hurt me the most was that my wife was refused the recommended afternoon treatment with the help of restorative assistants. The therapy department had said that she needed to walk twice a day to recover from her hip injury. Now she had another setback. It was an unfortunate accident, but it would greatly affect her ability to recover completely from her hip fracture. Exercise is very important, the more the better; ask anyone who has had a hip fracture.

CHAPTER THIRTEEN

Determination

I was there every day, not once, but twice.

There was an LPN who could have helped her. She seemed to have a lot of time when men came to visit a patient and chatted with them extensively. And even after she did her required work, she sat and talked to other employees. Both shifts had to be on the floor before the exchange of duties began. First, the two charge nurses exchanged information with each other. Then the charge nurse of the new shift talked to her nurses, and her last meeting was with the nursing assistants. After this meeting was over, they did not go to work but stayed in the room and killed time. Then they had to go to the supply room and load up their carts with supplies to do their shifts. It could take up to forty minutes to start their jobs.

Some of the staff had everything ready to go after the exchange meeting and went to work right away. This attitude died after the management changed to corporate ways of treating their employees. If you do not treat your employees well and consider them as second-class persons or as commodities that can be replaced just as easy as a tool, you cannot expect them to perform at their best. You need to give them respect for the demanding job they do. If you don't pay them the money they should receive to support a family, then they will not be committed to their patients. Who can support a family on eight or ten dollars an hour and have to pay for childcare? The nursing-home industry could not function properly without the nursing assistants and the kitchen and laundry help. Even if these are all entry-level jobs, they are the foundation on which the nursing-home industry depends. Only a good, strong foundation will support the structure. There are too many chiefs, too much paperwork, too much food wasted, and too much time wasted in meetings and training sessions, which do not improve care. At best, some cosmetic changes are implemented, but they do not alter the existing conditions. In this day and age, all medical records and administrative data should be on the computer. While I was thinking about all these problems, it suddenly dawned on me that my wife fell early in the morning. I was not even at the nursing home. I was called at home when she was supposed to be in bed. I was called when they were walking her. Why this early? It was always done after I was present and she was washed and dressed. I found out the names of the two assistants who were with her when this happened. In the afternoon, I raised that question with Danny and asked him what he could find out.

Christina stayed in bed. I cranked her bed down to a lower position. These beds were very old, and if you wanted to raise them, you had to hand crank them. The rails on the sides had to be pulled up by hand. I talked to her and held her hands. Suddenly, she bent forward and put her lips forward in a round position. When I saw this I kissed her and put my arms around her. I always kissed her when I came and left, but to me this was an expression of appreciation. It did not last long. I got tears in my eyes and knew this as one of those very rare moments that she really knew for a very short time that I was still with her and cared for her.

The next day I was surprised to find out that my wife had her own recliner. After we washed and dressed her, I pushed the recliner up and down the halls. Then I remembered that the cover of the cushion was shiny and so was the material of the chair. I needed friction to stop this. So I asked, "What do you do to stop her from sliding down?"

"You need a frog."

"What's that?"

"It is an anti-slip material; put it under her and it will not slide again."

"Where can I get this?"

"You have to request it."

I went to the charge nurse and explained what was going on with my wife in the recliner. "Please, could you order a piece of that anti-slip material for her? It is so uncomfortable for her to sit in that position," I asked.

"Yes I will order that for her."

A day went by and nothing happened, then another day, so I asked again. I was told, "I will check into it," but nothing happened. This made me upset. *Why should my wife sit in such an awkward position?* If you see your grandchild sitting like that, you will pull him up. It is a terrible sight, but if you do not care, you ignore the sight. *What is wrong with some of the nursing staff?* I had seen this material from other patients on her floor who had it. It was cut from a larger piece. It was similar to material that you put under a small rug, but I never knew that this would be used in nursing homes. On my way home, I passed a store that sold this material and explained that I did not need this for a rug but for my wife, because the nursing home she was in was very slow in supplying this to my wife. He sold me a medium size, which I took home and cut into different squares. I expected that one might disappear. These cushions were called "frogs," and it took some time before the frogs became part of the standard nursing-home supplies. They looked better than my homemade ones. They had a border around them, and on each corner strings to tie the piece down.

One afternoon, I entered my wife's room. She woke up and I kissed and talked to her. When the nursing assistant came in to check her and get ready for the afternoon, I looked for the recliner, but it was not in the room. I asked, "Where is the recliner?"

She told me that the charge nurse had told another aide to take the recliner and use it for another patient. When I heard her name, it clicked instantly. The charge nurse and the patient were from the same European background. I had noticed before that this patient got better treatment if the nurse was on duty. I went to her and asked, "Why did you use my wife's chair for her?"

"Doctor's orders."

This made me furious. I knew that a doctor would not do this. He would not sign an order to take the recliner away from my wife and give it to another patient. So I said to her, "Please show me the doctor's order." When she did not respond, I asked her to return the recliner to my wife. She did not do it, and I walked to the nurses' station and requested that the supervisor on duty come and see me. When she came, I explained the whole situation to her. She listened to me and said, "I will be back."

It took some time, but she came back with a recliner that was newer and better than the one we had before. I expressed my thanks and appreciation. As a general rule, supervisors do a pretty good job in a "no-win" situation. I have great respect for them. All the problems of the nursing home are dumped in their laps, including the chronic shortage of medical personnel and urgent medical problems.

I was home—it was past 9:00 p.m.—when I got a call from the nursing home. My wife had received medication that had not been intended for her. In other words, the nurse had made a mistake. How was this possible? She had her bracelet with her name on it, and if she was already in bed, her name was in large letters on the headboard, facing anybody entering the room. It was clearly visible to anyone assigned to give medication. After the nurse found out what she had done, she reported this to the charge nurse, who took action. The nurse who made this mistake was pulled from another floor because of a shortage of LPNs on this floor. I knew that whenever this happened, the nurse that was pulled away from her own floor was upset and in a bad mood. The charge nurse told me that nothing could be done about the high-blood-pressure medication, but for the insulin medication, they were feeding her a lot of ice cream, which apparently she seemed to enjoy. I was very upset and made up my mind to put this event in writing to the nursing-home administrator.

I did not sleep much that night. All the bad memories from wrong medications my wife had received in the past came back to mind. I wrote the complaint, and the next morning, I handed it over for processing by the nursing home. It took some time before the administrator called me in to talk about this incident. The administrator knew that I was a daily visitor. He called me during a visit to make an appointment with him at a time convenient to both of us.

On that day, after my morning visit, I went to his office and told his secretary that I was here for an appointment. After the formalities, I started to explain what had happened to my wife on that particular evening, receiving medication that was not for her, but for another patient. He did not go into any detail, but defended the LPN, saying that she was a good worker. He did not apologize for her or the fact that this had happened. He would not let the LPN make an apology, which I would have appreciated very much. I do not have any bad feelings about them. I see daily what they have to endure. In fact, I am more on their side than in agreement with the administrator. Then he changed the subject and complimented me on my dedication to be with my wife and said, "I hope that my wife will do the same for me."

We were just exchanging words without any real purpose. I closed the conversation with the remark that I did not want to see this LPN on my wife's floor when the nursing home ran short of LPNs. I was not really surprised about the outcome of the conversation. He was not only defending his job, but also upholding the status quo of the nursing-home industry, where the bottom line is profit and care or quality of care is somehow low the list of objectives. They carefully walk the line between negligence and mediocre care. In the nursing home, it is true that in the land of the blind, the one-eyed person is in charge.

We had a new activity director who believed that music was good medicine. In order to please the residents as much as possible, she played different kinds of music. One day she brought in a Yamaha player and played "I Could Have Danced All Night." I was sitting close to Christina when suddenly the upper part of her body started to make dancing movements, just as if we were dancing. She had been a better dancer than I. This lasted only a short time. The slow dying of her brain took even these short moments of remembrance and joy away from her. These events occurred after music was played or when we rested from our strolls to take in a change of scenery. This time, she said in our native language, "You are a very good husband." I knew that she was very secure about my care and compassion for her. I would not abandon her, but would do everything in my power to undo the neglect of the nursing-home industry and to provide the best care for her, as all citizens should have in their old age.

Christina had one more surprise for the staff and me. Sometimes when she was in her recliner, she started to laugh, sometimes very loudly. If I was not present, the staff reported to me that she had been laughing again. That peace of mind was beyond our understanding.

It was a constant worry to keep Christina clean and dry. You do not know this unless you do what I do and look under the blankets. This is the only way to know. I made sure my wife was clean as long as I was there. All I could do was hope for the best in the other hours that I was not present. In twenty-four hours, I was with her between five and six hours each day. The remainder of that time, my wife depended on the staff and their commitment and compassion. Most of them did the best they could, even though the management did not appreciate their dedication, which was the nurses' biggest complaint. By appreciation, I do not mean the occasional treats by supervisors at national holidays or free meals at religious events. The corporate spirit does not have "appreciation for employees" as one of their business objectives; their bottom line is money.

One evening after I left the floor, I met a supervisor. He had worked for many years as a charge nurse in a large hospital. When he retired from there, he came to work for the nursing home. He had helped me in the past and I appreciated not only his knowledge but also his friendship. That evening, I approached him with my problem of the madman on the Alzheimer's floor. I told him what had happened and what the staff had told me about this man. We talked for some time and he advised me to go to the nursing-home administrator. I did not tell him about my first unproductive encounter with the administrator.

My meeting with Brad, the nursing-home administrator, started with the conventional remarks, and then I started to tell him that I wanted the madman, Henry, transferred to another floor. There are many forms you have to fill out and sign upon admittance to the nursing home. One of them states that if a person does harm to himself or others, he can be removed from the facility. He did harm to my wife to such an extent that she broke her hip and underwent surgery. She was not the only one he had hurt. I was certain about that.

"What shall I tell his family?" was Brad's response.

"Why do you ask me this? You are in charge. You know you can make decisions yourself." I suggested a compromise. "Can you instruct the staff on this floor to move the row of chairs in the hall to another location? This area is so congested with people walking or standing near the nurses' station, it is not safe for the patients." (He did not respond to this request. But years later when I visited this unit again, I was really surprised to see that what I mentioned at that meeting had indeed been done. In fact, it looked better than any other floor in the building, with no chairs clogging essential traffic areas.) I continued and told him, "This man has not hurt once but several times; he is a repeat offender."

"What shall I say to his family?"

"You know what is in that admissions form. Why do you keep him on that floor? You do not hear complaints from other visitors because they do not see or hear about it. I am one of the few who come in daily so I know more about what is going on each day. Accidents are recorded with no name of the perpetrator. This man endangers the safety not only of the patients but also of the staff. He is extremely strong. He uses his arms as weapons. One female nurse cannot handle him; only the male nurse can do this. You seem to be more concerned about the man's family. What about the victim's families? Is it okay because they do not know or are not told? Why don't you move him off this floor? Tell his family in a nice way that it is better for him to go to another floor where there are not so many patients walking. If this had happened outside, I could have called the police to file a complaint against this man. He would have been liable for my wife's hip fracture and could be arrested." No matter what I said, he would not take any action against this man.

I told the nurses' assistants that I had a dental appointment and could not be on time to help them the next morning. When I arrived after my appointment the next day, Christina was already dressed and in her recliner, but there was no support for her legs, and her body was too close to one side. I needed help to adjust her position. I kissed her and said, "I will get some help." She was in a small area where at the most three recliners could be parked, with a chair for me to sit next to her. I returned to my wife, put my jacket on the back of her recliner, took a chair and sat down. When an LPN passed, I asked her to help me adjust Christina's posture in the chair. She was no longer able to sit in a chair without bending forward and slouching sideways. I corrected this by using her bed pillows. She had her eyes open and seemed to look in the direction of sound she could hear. I remembered seeing people in wheelchairs. Their bodies bent over to the side and also forward. I had not forgotten that terrible sight. *What dignity is left? A nation that does not care for their elderly is a nation without compassion.*

I had a snack for Christina; it was vanilla custard pudding. I started to feed her, but she was very slow in accepting each spoonful. Then I smelled poop. One of the patients stopped and started talking to me. Another was heading with her walker for the chair next to me, and when she sat down, she asked, "When do I go home?" The standard answer from the staff was always four o'clock, so that is what I told her; another answer might have upset her.

"Your wife is a beautiful woman. Is she getting better?"

"No."

"What a shame. I was born in the United States, but I am Italian. Does she like it here?"

"No."

"Do you want to go back?"

"Yes, if I could."

My wife would not eat anymore and closed her eyes. I smelled poop again. I pushed her out the waiting room and parked her in a safe location and asked the charge nurse if she could call Ruth and Mary, the nursing assistants, because Christina needed to be changed. The charge nurse went down the hall and called and looked in the rooms, but no answer. Then she went to the dayroom to see if they were there, but they were not there, either. It was close to break time. The nurse returned to her desk. Where were those two nursing assistants? I knew if she were not cleaned now, they would let her sit in that soft stool. After waiting five minutes, which seemed like a half hour to me, I went back to the nurse and repeated my request. A short time later, one of the assistants came, pushing the manual lift in the direction of my wife's room. I followed her with the recliner. The linen cart was in the hall, so I went to it and took out underpads, towels, and washcloths. I put these on the end of her bed and went to her cabinet to get clean clothes. While I was getting supplies from the linen cart, the other aide came down the hall and asked, "Did you see Ruth?"

"Yes, my wife is in the room. I have all the things you need to clean her. The lift placed her in bed and they removed the sling and started to clean her. Ruth said, "I need more underpads," so I went out and got two more. When I came back, Ruth's gloves were so soiled that she needed clean ones. Each room had a container with gloves so I pulled a pair out and handed them to her. The soft stool had spread to the lower part of her stomach, in between her legs and into her buttocks. I held her hands so she would not scratch and put her hands in the soft stool. It took quite a while to get her clean, and I decided to keep her in bed until the afternoon. They also put cream on all the irritated skin. When they were done, it was twenty minutes past their break time.

"I really appreciate what you have done. Thank you very much."

Ruth told me that Christina was up very early that morning. If she stayed in bed, she might eat better. Yesterday they checked her about the same time and she was soaking wet. I was really touched by the loving care of those dedicated nursing assistants. It was a good feeling to see this compassion at work. Believe me, it is not an easy job to clean my wife under these conditions.

One morning, my wife was in bed, and I saw that her cheeks were red. It could be that there were too many covers on her. It was also very hot in the room, so I removed one cover. Then I put down the guard rail and sat down and stroked her cheeks when Jan came in. "We did not know if you wanted her up, so we waited until you came. It is better to keep her in bed." Another nursing assistant came, and while I was stroking my wife's cheeks, she put her hand my shoulder. "I know; I took care of my mother for four years. You are just as sweet as she was." Another came in and told us that she had attended a football game at the high school last night. It reminded me of our daughter, who was in the high school band. They played and marched and played and marched. Christina and I used to take blankets and hot coffee to stay warm when we watched her at the football game. Then the assistant checked my wife. She was dry, but had a loose stool. "I will change that. Her skin is looking pretty good, but yesterday and the day before, her buttocks were inflamed and some places looked dark red. It looks that way when the urine and bowel movement stay too long on her skin. The ointment will take care of that." I assisted her, holding my wife on her side and rolling her over to the other side to get her clean and put the ointment on again. I bent over my wife and said, "She is a nice lady. She takes good care of you and quite a few others, too." I took her hands and watched her. She had her eyes closed. Emotions came up and became stronger until my eyes were filled with tears.

One morning when we were sitting out in the hall, Christina was sleeping and I was holding her hand. A physical therapist walked behind me and whispered in my ear, "I wish somebody would love me as much as you love your wife." The night shift charge nurse was a straight shooter, and I had heard a lot about her. One morning, she stayed on for the first shift and walked past us and said, "Where do I find a man like that? I would like to have one like that."

The staff social worker was extremely diplomatic. She approached me when I was pushing my wife up and down the hall. "I hear you are very concerned about your wife's safety on this floor, and we share that concern. We would like to help to solve this problem. Would you consider moving her to another floor? We have three immediate openings, and two more are coming up soon." My answer was very short. "It is not my wife who is making the trouble.

What is so special about this man that he can't be transferred?" She did not answer, but flashed a nice smile to end the conversation.

When December came around again, I had to recruit volunteers to help with the Christmas meal for our floor. So far, our church members had done pretty well. I was now attending two support meetings. The first one was the Alzheimer's association, and the second one was the nursing-home group. They met once a month. I began attending the association meeting when my wife was still at home. One man who came to our meeting told how he was in charge of his mother's money. He visited her twice a week and attended the monthly support meeting. He never told us why he was the only one who visited her. He was one of eleven children, and his mother was a person who seemed to be in command and always got what she wanted. This was clear in her relationship with her friends at the nursing home. When confrontations took place, she always came out ahead. The staff never witnessed what happened in that small room. The son always brought up the subject that no one from the family visited their mother. It was good that he could talk about it. At this year's Christmas party, he got a big surprise. The man from the support was not alone this time. Eight-eight members of his family showed up! Brothers, sisters, spouses, children, grandchildren and a few great-grandchildren. This was the best Christmas he ever had in his life. It was the number-one talk of the nursing home for quite some time.

One morning I came and Christina was in bed, which was not unusual, but she had company. Another patient was in the bed next to Christina's bed. I walked to Christina's side and looked at her. What was surprising was that Christina looked at the woman in the bed next to hers and started to laugh really loud. The woman's eyes opened up, and Christina kept on laughing, but not as loud. I kissed Christina twice. She never looked that long at me. It was always a short time. I kissed her more than once. She did not go into that unconscious state. I kissed her more. Then she started to make sounds as if she was talking. There were no words, just sounds. She kept doing this and kept looking at me and looked very happy. These moments were great rewards. The fact that I could share this great time with her meant a lot to me. How many people miss opportunities like this when they do not visit their loved ones? She still had a happy expression on her face even after she stopped laughing. I put her in my arms and held her tight. I held her for quite some time. Then she closed her eyes and started to lean. I put her down, watched her, and held her hand.

I realized that they were late this morning and wondered why. I knew they would come sooner or later, so I took her clothes out of her closet. I went to the linen cart and took all that was needed to get her washed and dressed and put the items on her bed. Sharon, one of the assistants, came into the room. "I am a little late on my schedule."

"I brought in all you need from the linen cart and her clothes."

"Oh. I left the soap bottle in the other room; I will get it." When she came back, Kelly was with her. They started to get my wife ready. I told them what had happen just a short time ago, that she laughed and stayed alert much longer than at other times, but then she closed her eyes. They were quite talkative that morning. Sharon told me that she had given a back rub to a resident who seemed to like it very much. She mentioned that her mother had a boyfriend. Kelly told me in detail how she was feeding squirrels who came to her window, jumping from tree branches to the gutter. She was trying to gain their trust and feed them. I told them about the problems I had with rabbits and squirrels. In the spring, the mother rabbit came to our lawn, dug a hole, and used it only as a maternity ward. After that, she transferred the little ones to another spot. The squirrels would do the same damage. First they buried the nuts from the tree in the lawn, and in spring time they would visit their storage area and leave holes all over our yard. "I know we took their farm land, but why do they like our lawn better than our neighbors'?"

Christina did not have a bowel movement and was only wet after washing. They put lotion on her back, legs, and feet. They put cream on her buttocks, rolled her from left to right, from right to left, dressed her, put the cotton sling under her and transferred her to the recliner. I rolled her to our spot next to the window at the end of the hall.

I tried to give her the pudding, but she was not too eager to eat and closed her eyes again. I held her hand and she gave a big sigh. She did this a lot lately. Then I saw Pollyanna coming; she was alone this time. She walked quietly up to the window and looked outside for some time. Then she turned around and started to talk. "My brother and I were standing at this window and were looking at the sky. It was a clear night. I felt so peaceful and content. Now this morning, it is so beautiful when the sun rises, especially in this part. You see all kinds of colors. It is such a nice state. I hope I can stay here for a long time. You probably will be going too, but what about your wife? Only the Lord knows. It gives you a good feeling," she put her hand on her chest and then on her head. "It is so good to talk to you. Most people do not talk about this. They are probably afraid to show their feelings. It is good to talk with you."

CHAPTER FOURTEEN

Assets

The Robert Wood Johnson Foundation came up with good partnership plans to protect the assets of persons who would require long-term care and reduce each state's Medicaid budget.

Dollar for Dollar Approach

You buy a partnership-certified policy, which is different in each state. The policyholder receives from Medicaid a dollar of protection of his or her assets for every dollar the insurance company spends for his or her long-term care insurance. For example, Mr. Jones has total assets of $150,000. He purchases a state-certified long-term care insurance policy with a maximum paid-out value of $150,000. If Mr. Jones needs long-term care, the insurance company pays the daily benefits to the nursing home. When the policy finishes paying all the benefits, Mr. Jones goes on Medicaid. He keeps his $150,000. His income will continue to go to the nursing home. His spouse at home is allowed her share of the income.

Complete Assets Approach

This works differently in each state. You need to buy a partnership-certified long-term care insurance policy that pays for at least three years of nursing-home care at a minimum of one hundred dollars a day, or six years of home health care at fifty dollars a day or a combination of both.

When the policy has paid all the benefits, he or she will be eligible for Medicaid and their assets of $100,000 will be protected. His or her income will go to the nursing home, and the spouse at home is allowed his or her share of the income.

ONLY ELEVEN STATES WERE ABLE TO PUT THIS PARTNERSHIP INTO LAW. AFTER THE DEADLINE, NO PERMISSION WAS GRANTED BY THE HEALTH-CARE FINANCING ADMINSTRATION.

What went wrong? The Robert Wood Johnson Foundation has studied the long-term care problem in regard to the ability to pay for these costs. If long-term care were included in regular health insurance policies, the cost would be shared by the victims of this disease, their spouses, and the state. It would not punish the middle class for saving money, but come up with plan to protect their assets and pay their fair share.

We listen too much to television and radio. The media did not provide us with both sides of the health-care issue. It was a one-way street of information. We heard and read about Medicare reform day-in, day-out for weeks, for months, always working on our fear that the corporate insurance companies would be much better than national health care. No health-care system is perfect. Each one of them has its faults, but with corporate health care, the bottom line is profit, not patient satisfaction. National health care would provide coverage for every citizen. Corporate health care leaves the poor and the needy unprotected. We have over thirty million citizens who do not have health care and that is not only a great shame but also in violation of the Human Rights Bill. Our country signed this bill. Do we have the courage to call our Congressmen, the government violators of Human Rights, and point this out to them? The lawmakers we elected seem to listen more to the lobbyists who supply them with lots of money for their reelection.

Ralph Nader's organization has printed a list of all the elected officials who are on the payroll of the corporations. Get it and read it. We used to have a media that provided us with both sides of any issue, but that does not exist anymore. Mergers and buyouts narrowed down competition, not only in the industrial sections but in all sections of our economy. The news media was part of this concentration of power in the management of a few large corporations. It did not take long before most Democratic party-owned media were forced to sell or merge with Republican-owned news conglomerates. They make the news we hear a one-way street by omitting facts or producing facts to justify corporate goals.

The biggest and most destructive myths the media heaped upon us created much doubt and fear, telling us that national health care would not allow us to select our own doctors, that it would be managed by government bureaucrats who would tell us what kinds of treatment we could have, tell us what kinds of drugs we were allowed to have access to, and create an enormous amount of paperwork. It would raise our premium in social security tax.

The public relations corporations were hired by the insurance industry and did the job they were paid for, and we all fell for it. We were told that the private sector of insurance could do a much better job. We were not told that thirty million citizens would be excluded. We did not even know that we were brainwashed. Brainwashing is not new. It is an old tool that has been used throughout the ages.

The public relations corporations also worked on members of Congress with the usual monetary rewards. All we heard on TV, on the radio, and in newspapers were lies. It was the HMOs (health maintenance organizations) who did not allow us to select the doctors we wanted. We were buried under all the new forms from each HMO, not the standard form but many, many, many different forms. The free-market story was a joke; it did not work. Costs went up, services were cut, and quality went down. Doctors were told by the insurance companies to cut costs by refusing to refer people to specialists and were rewarded for this negligence. The compensation for CEOs in the insurance industry reached an all-time high. Incompetent CEOs were given compensation that was unbelievably high. Profits soared.

Reaching a person at an HMO is time consuming. The recorded voice tells you to make a selection from a list. If your topic is not on the list, you are told to wait for the next available customer service representative.

The Omnibus Reconciliation Act of 1993 was a violation of Article 25 of the Universal Declaration of Human Rights. It specifies that the estate of anyone dying after October 1, 1993, is subject to medical recovery. Virtually all programs designed for low-income families would be eliminated and replaced with state block grants, which could be lowered. Rather than reforming the system to make it more efficient, Congress instead has plotted to cut medical coverage to the needy as a way of balancing the federal budget.

This backward approach had significant impact on the elderly in the areas of nursing-home care and the cutting of home care services. This budget cut in many ways targets the less fortunate, those on welfare, and the middle class. The elderly would be enticed to transfer their benefits from Supplement B to HMO benefits, which would be less. Medical doctors would not be allowed to tell which benefits were excluded. There would be a rate set for reimbursing daily nursing-home care. This rate would lower the quality of care or result in closing this kind of care. When this act had to be applied, not too many knew how to interpret it. It took quite some time before anyone could make sense of it.

The pharmaceutical industry came up with Tacrine, the first drug approved by the FDA for treatment of Alzheimer's, in 1993. The second, Donepezil, came in 1996, and in 1999 they approved the third drug, to become available in 2000, Rivastigmine.

Alzheimer's is not a natural result of aging. It is over diagnosed by about twenty-five percent by doctors. The process of elimination of other illness would allow them to say, "It is not this; it is not that, so it has to be Alzheimer's." It has nothing to do with your IQ. It strikes rich and poor, women, men, and young adults. No race is excluded.

The nursing-home social worker approached me one day. She started to talk about almost everything, but then suddenly changed the subject: "I am afraid your wife will be transferred to another floor." No other explanation was given. Had this to do with my request to transfer the madman and she was sent to tell me? I knew that I needed professional help and told her, "I will talk to our attorney about this."

At a support group meeting from the Alzheimer's Association, a lawyer who specialized in this kind of law had given us a brief overview on how to protect our assets when our spouse or parent had to go to a nursing home. I had his name and telephone number.

I called his office and made an appointment. The office was downtown, a section well kept up in a two hundred year old town. A small park was across the street. Street parking was available if you did not come at rush hour. The hall was large, with windows big enough that no electric lights were needed in that area. The receptionist called the lawyer and informed him of my arrival. I was told that coffee was available in a small room across the hall. I was also given a copy of a typed letterhead, listing all the partners with their specialized field and their fees, which were in the three-digit range. I was scared looking at these amounts.

I told this attorney everything that had happened to my wife in the nursing home. The hip fracture, the madman, the care that you have to monitor by being present, my visits twice a day, the nursing assistants who had to get used to me and helped me, how I talked with the nursing-home administrator and the licensed staff, the housekeepers, and kitchen staff.

I told him that we had used our savings to pay for her care, which our Congress called "spending down." He was familiar with this nursing home and the new laws. He knew the federal and state laws and the nursing homes rules and regulations, which at that time made him an expert in elderly law. We could fight this problem, but it would be costly to win. The down-spending of our savings was for the nursing home. Up to this point, Christina was classified as a private patient, but when this stopped, she would be transferred to Medicaid. It would be normal business to transfer my wife to a Medicaid bed. The empty bed on the unit would be available for another patient who could afford to pay private fees until their time came and then they would be transferred.

I told the attorney that I had learned through the grapevine in the nursing home that this was not always true. He acknowledged this. I did not want to create feelings that might influence the quality of care my wife received. I was there for many hours, but not twenty-four hours. I would like to keep the friendly association I had with the majority of the nursing assistants and the licensed staff. I told the attorney that I would talk to the nursing-home administrator and keep his offer to help for another time.

I asked for an appointment with the administrator after my morning visit, which I did get. I explained to her that my wife and I had many friends on this unit. It took years to establish these relationships. If she was transferred, we would miss this little spark of hope and comfort.

"Christina knows and feels more than we generally assume. It is just like a person in a coma who hears a voice and feels the touch and these little expressions of love, care, and compassion. A transfer will emotionally harm her; adjusting to a new staff will do no good." The administrator listened as I continued, "I remember one day when she was recovering from the hip fracture, caused by a patient on her floor, a woman came into her room. She saw the white sheets and me sitting next to Christina, holding her hand; she made the sign of the cross as she was kneeling and started to pray. I could not understand her, she spoke Spanish. Then she stood up and touched her hands, spoke a few words and left the room talking to herself."

The administrator nodded as I kept talking. "After supper, patients come from the day room and ask me, 'How is she?' When she is alert I respond, 'She is doing okay today.' At other times, when she is in pain, when her eyes are closed, I respond, 'She is not doing so well.' They say, 'There is not much that we can do, but we will pray for her.' When they come and her eyelids are closed, they say, 'We will pray a little harder.'

"There is another woman who comes into the room, puts her hand on my shoulder, points to my wife, and says, 'She is very pretty.' Then she tells me that somebody came in her house and took a lot of money. I ask, 'Did you report this to the police?' She keeps on talking about other things. I first met this woman when I was pushing my wife in the recliner, before the accident. I stopped and smiled at her and she responded with a smile. Then I put my hand on her shoulder and she remained quiet for some time."

The administrator asked me why I had asked for this meeting

"You let the man push my wife and she broke her hip; he is still a threat to all patients on the floor, but you do not transfer him."

"Oh, I do not remember that."

"But you want to transfer her? It will do her no good. Adjusting takes a long time; when she came here, it took almost a year. All the patients on this unit will miss us. Please let her stay."

Two weeks later, my wife was transferred to another floor. Through the grapevine, I heard that the social worker had resigned. She had found a much better nursing home to work in.

I would not abandon my wife. I would make sure she would be taken care of as long as there was breath in me.

CHAPTER FIFTEEN

The Hospice

In the winter of 2001, when I came out of the elevator, there were several strange people in front of the nurses' station. This was quite unusual. I did not pay much attention, but it was not the normal routine. There were people there I had never seen before. One of the staff told me that it was the state inspector and his colleagues. I went to my wife's room. Kelly came into the room and told me that one of the aides had reported Christina's condition to the inspector. Soon after that, the state inspector came to Christina's room, and when he saw her condition, he took action. She also told me that the front patient rooms, closest to the nurses' station, were "paying" rooms. We had lost all our life savings for Christina's care and we were now in the rooms paid for by the state. The inspector visited these rooms last. The inspector's visit was at 10 a.m. By 12 p.m., Christina was on her way to the hospice. As soon as the hospice nurse had heard what the doctor had said, she walked out of the room to call her office. She set the transfer in motion, called an ambulance, and told me it would take about forty-five minutes to get to the hospice. The doctor put the nursing staff into action as I had never seen before in all my years at the nursing home. Flying was not the right word, but it came pretty close.

I went back to my wife's room and went to her closet and took the few things she had and packed them. I left Christina's two hand-knit covers for the staff. Her nightstand did not contain much, either; it only had socks. I took the socks as she would need them in the hospice to keep her feet warm. I asked the nurses for a plastic bag so I could pack up the radio, the small electric fan, a thermometer, and a pillow that I had brought from home. It was a pillow from our bed at home, a large queen size. I looked at Christina and took her hands; they were warm. Her lips were not closed, but her eyes were. The skin covering her head had taken the shape of the skull, because all the underlying tissue had disappeared. Emotions bubbled in me; tears came to my eyes.

"You will get out of this place. No more forced feeding, no more choking. The staff misused your friendly nature. You did not slap their hands; you could not. It took time to feed you. Only a few tried, the best, but chronic shortages day in, day out made your life miserable. From now on, you do not have to eat anymore against your will. You are now free from the nursing-home industry rules. You are going to a place where compassion, not the money to keep the shareholders happy, is number one. I will go with you and continue to care for you as I did here for seven years. I also know you will die there. I heard that you cannot live for more than seven days without food or water." I took my lip balm and rubbed it on her lips as I had done for many years, day in, day out, every morning, every afternoon. Then I watched her. The social worker arrived. She never knocked on the door. She was one who thought rules did not apply to her. She showed me a paper that I had to sign, but she misspelled my name so I made her fix it.

It would take about forty-five minutes for the ambulance to arrive. This would give me plenty of time to bring the few worldly possessions Christina had to the car. This morning, I was quite early because I had counted on feeding her. At that time, there were plenty of parking spaces in front of the building. When I placed the plastic bag in the back of our car, an ambulance pulled up in front of the building. This was not unusual; it happens all the time. The attendants pulled out the litter and brought it inside. When I came in the hall, they were waiting.

One elevator is reserved for emergencies, and a guard stands watch so that no one uses it. It suddenly dawned on me that this litter was for my wife. The attendants were waiting for that elevator and I rode up with them. When we got to Christina's room, they raised the litter to the level of the bed. I removed the Foley catheter from the side and put it on the bed. The pillow from her contracted leg was removed and she was lifted from the air mattress to the hard mattress of the litter, and it must have hurt her. I put the pillow back between her legs so she would be comfortable during transport. I also took the pillow at the head of the bed, since it was from our home and was longer and more comfortable for her. They strapped this pillow to the litter. I also made sure that the air mattress would be brought to the hospice. We left the room and waited in front of the elevators to go down. A few staff members said, "Good-bye," and one hugged me. It was pretty cold that morning and the hospice nurse said, "She must be cold with that thin cover," but the pillow on her body gave her some protection. My wife was placed inside the ambulance. After the door was closed, I walked to our car but remembered that I had left a plastic bag on the floor, so I had to go back and get it. When I came back, the ambulance was gone. I drove to the hospice center.

It was a short drive from the east end of town through the downtown area and then the reconstruction zone of the highway. The reconstruction had been going on for three years now and would probably not be complete for another two years in this rapidly expanding western section of the city. In this part of town, they had already built a large medical center, which was an extension of the downtown hospital. It housed all the new medical equipment. This latest building was just for mothers and babies. The doctors had built a large building to house their offices. It was at the edge of this very large medical development that a small hospice building was constructed. Close to the highway, you could see the traffic but not hear the noise. From the outside, it did not look like a hospital, nursing home, or doctor's building. The large hallway entrance had only one desk. The volunteer behind it directed me to the office. Here I was told where my wife was. Walking toward this room, I got the feeling I was in a home, a very tastefully decorated home. There were large grandfather clocks, wall-to-wall carpeting with lovely patterns, lots of windows with drapes, and some with stained glass. The exterior was beautifully landscaped. I passed a room with a fireplace, and the numbers on the room doors were painted on ceramic tiles. I came to the end of the hall and there was Christina's room. I knocked on the door, which was ajar, and stepped inside. There she was lying on her own mattress, her eyes closed, mouth open. There were two nurses in the room and they introduced themselves. They told me that the ambulance attendants had set up the air mattress and the control unit. This was quite a change. In the nursing home, they were not quite as efficient. This air mattress replaces the work of the nurses, who have to turn the patient from side to side every two hours. The mattress does the job. Our children had purchased this rotating mattress for their mother to prevent bed sores. The nursing-home industry may talk about the dangers of bed sores and their attempt to prevent them, but that's where it stops. The staff never seems to have time to take care of the basic needs of the patients, let alone turn them every two hours. As long as relatives do not care for or take part in the care of their elderly family members confined to a nursing home, this national crisis will continue. There are relatives who only visit on holidays. Others do not come at all or just phone in. Most ministers shy away from nursing homes. *It's the people at the end of their lives that need the attention and comfort.* The baby boomers are too busy with their retirement portfolios and watching the stock market. They do not speak up for the ones who cannot speak for themselves.

Driving home, I suddenly started to cry. This day had been too much for me. I was on emotional overload.

The next day when I arrived, I noticed that my wife had only one blanket on her bed. I touched the material and it felt light. I asked the nurse for another blanket. She brought two. The nurse removed the sheet and blanket from Christina and placed the new blanket over her body and feet then replaced the sheet and blanket. I was very happy about this; it showed good care. The other blanket was left in the room. This was a private room with a nightstand and lamp on either side of the bed. There was also a radio/CD player on the left nightstand. The nurse asked if I had photos of Christina. I had two photos, one of our wedding day and one of Christina in her nurse's uniform. My wife had made her own wedding gown in Amsterdam with fabric from Paris. She was an excellent seamstress, very attentive to detail and finishing. It took her a year to finish this gown. The nurse asked if I could display the photos. I said yes and we put them in the corners of the frame of the painting that was hanging over her bed. The social worker came in and introduced herself. The nurse said, "Look at her pictures."

After some time, I took the other blanket and put it over Christina while holding her hands. A nurse came in and brought some CDs from the Hospice Center. The nurse showed me how to use the CD player, and I played a CD I thought Christina would enjoy. No reaction on her face, but I was sure that she felt my hand and heard some sound. I had played tapes for her in the nursing home, usually during the second shift. I was more at peace here at the hospice. I was content with the good care she was getting and the relief that we no longer had to force-feed her. I'm sure we both shared this sense of peace and comfort. I held her hands and they were now warm, so we kept them under the blankets. I also had to tell the hospice nurses that she needed two pairs of socks. One regular pair, then over those, the fleece Toasties with the anti-slip strips on the bottom. It was routine in the nursing home to take the socks off the patients' feet, but I had instructed them to keep Christina's on, and now I had to tell the hospice nurses the same.

There were two chairs and a small table in the sitting area of Christina's room. Two of the walls had windows, one looking out to the yard. This window had a built-in bench with pillows. The other wall was at a right angle to the patio door, which was the French type. The blind wall was shared with the next room. If you sat up in bed, you could watch the traffic on the highway, but you could not hear the sound of cars. I placed one of the chairs on the left side of the bed and I saw that it was time to moisten her lips. Then I noticed that on the other nightstand was a small container of Vaseline, and in it was a Q-tip with a long handle. I pulled the handle out to see if there was enough on the swab to coat her lips. This worked much better than the lip balm I always used. From that moment on, I did not use lip balm anymore.

Christina did not react at all anymore. I was, however, very happy with the caring staff here, and I did not feel nervous leaving her to go home and get some rest or have a meal. I knew she would be taken care of here with compassion and dignity.

I took my midday break and returned to find Christina's hands and feet still warm. I put my jacket in the closet and reapplied some Vaseline to her lips. I selected a new CD to play and made a mental note to bring some CDs from home. The shifts were different in the hospice center. There were no nurses' aides, only LPNs and RNs. None of these nurses had the urgency in their daily routine to care for more patients than was humanly possible. At the hospice, there were two staff members for each patient. Each private room had a large bathroom with a shower, a toilet, and a wall-to-wall vanity and sink. The cabinets of the vanity contained the medication (locked) and various medical supplies for the care of the hospice patient. There were no big, clunky carts wheeling down the hallway as there had been in the nursing home. All this was so different from the nursing-home industry, where patient care was dependent on meeting quotas. We are the richest country in the world, but when it comes to the general health care of all our citizens, we rank at the bottom. Out of the top thirteen free, industrialized countries, we rank twelfth. This is because we have thirty to fifty million citizens without health insurance.

If Christina's hands got cold, I took them in mine and rubbed them till they were warm, one at a time, and then placed the warmed hand on her body under the blanket. A nurse came in and I explained what I was doing. She asked me if I wanted coffee, and told me that there was a kitchen here that could be used to prepare meals. The nurse came back with the coffee and walked over to the bed to look at the photos of my wife. "They are nice," she said. "Yes she was only nineteen in her nurse's uniform and twenty-five in the wedding photo."

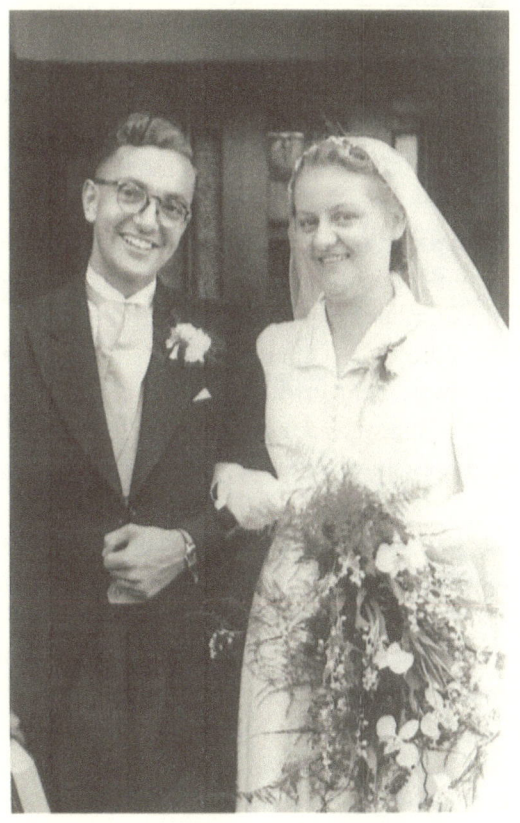

A woman entered the room and said she was a volunteer who came to the hospice once a month to play the dulcimer. I invited her in, since Christina loved music. Lucy brought in her stand first and put it at the end of the bed. She came in with the dulcimer and put it on the stand, took out two soft hammers, and hit the strings. It made a sweet tranquil sound. What Lucy played was not familiar to me, but it sounded excellent. Before she started a new piece she waited several moments, and then began a new piece. Later she started to play some hymns I knew. My wife was lying in bed, no change, but I kept her hands warm. After the recital, I asked about this instrument that makes happy sounds. Lucy explained that the name comes from the Latin "dulce" and the Greek "melos" which combined means "sweet tune." Its origin is the Near East, and has been played for about five thousand years. Much later, it traveled to China and Korea. It is the forerunner of the modern piano. The modern dulcimer has a shallow trapezoidal frame. The sound board has two bridges, which divide the top area into three sections. On the right is the bass bridge. To the left is the treble bridge. The bass string goes over the bass bridge and through a hole in the treble bridge to the other and over a side bridge to a pin, which is used for tuning. In the lumber camps of Michigan and Maine, the dulcimers were called "the Lumber Jack's piano." These dulcimers were plucked with the fingers and only had a few strings. They came in all sizes and shapes and were held in the lap while playing. The dulcimer is coming back in many places in Western Europe, and there is an explosion of interest in our country in using it for country, rock, and jazz music.

After Lucy left, the room was quiet again. My wife's hands and feet were still warm, so I went to the kitchen to get another cup of coffee. The first time I was there, I did not know which pot had the regular and which had the decaffeinated. The orange top was the decaffeinated. Drinking coffee in here was quite different from the nursing home, where in that long time I was only offered coffee twice. One my return to the room, I filled my glass with water, put the CD player on, sat down, and watched her respirations. She inhaled and exhaled very regularly. I did not count. Sometimes, it seemed as if Christina had stopped breathing. Or was that just the way it looked to me? I could not see her throat moving up or down. Did it stop or was the breath too shallow to notice? It would then start up rapidly and then go back to normal. On the first visit from the hospice center to determine if she would qualify for the program, the nurse told me that the lower part of her lungs did not work anymore. I was not surprised to hear this; the forced feeding must have allowed liquid to get into her lungs. How much she must have choked in these years could only be determined by an autopsy. I saw it only twice when I came in early during breakfast and later at lunch.

One morning, I had come into her room at the nursing home and the charge nurse was trying to get liquid out. She could not do it. She did not know how and my wife was suffering. I got very angry and told her to stop it. There was respiratory technician in the room and he asked me for permission to go through her nose. I said, "please as fast as you can." He did a good job, but in the meantime, my wife had unnecessarily suffered from the unprofessional help of the charge nurse. Suddenly these sad memories were interrupted when a hospice nurse came in to give Christina her medication. She went into the bathroom and unlocked the cabinet and prepared the pain medication for my wife.

In the nursing home I had to occasionally ask for more pain medication if Christina seemed to be in pain or discomfort. I was part of the daily routine there at the nursing home, so I could make requests for my wife, but what about the others who could not even use the call bell? Who would know if they were in pain if the nurses were not doing rounds at that time? It was not long after the first shift hospice nurse left that two more nurses entered the room and introduced themselves. They, too, wanted to see the pictures of my wife when she was young.

I wanted to leave the hospice that day before it got dark because I was not familiar the area. I kissed Christina good night, as I always did, checked her hands and feet. Then I took the coffee cup and glass to the kitchen and put them in the sink.

The next morning, even though her door was open, I knocked. My wife was lying to the extreme left side of the bed. I used the call bell and was surprised to get assistance so quickly. In the nursing-home industry, there are regulations and rules that each call bell has to be answered within a certain time limit. The reality with understaffing is different. Patients complain about this in meetings over and over again. Improvements are promised, but no real change will occur as long as there is a chronic shortage of nursing personnel. In the hospice, it was different. A nurse came right away and I explained what had to be done. She left the room and soon came back with another nurse to assist her.

The nurses in this hospice had never seen a mattress like Christina's. It replaced the work of the nurse by rolling the patient over onto her side, not by hand, but by inflating and deflating the sections of the mattress. The intervals could be set from fifteen minutes to an hour. I checked her hands; they were cold and her feet were warm. Her legs were cold. Why? Was it because of the position she was in? First, I put Vaseline on her lips and then got a glass of water and a cup of coffee from the kitchen. I put a CD into the player and pulled up a chair to the left side of the bed and started to warm her hands. I looked at her. There was no change. Her mouth was open, eyes closed. There was no body movement, but her hands were getting warmer. This always made me happy. I knew someday it would not be possible to warm her hands. I had brought a selection of CDs from our home.

Christina did not get any food or liquid. The doctor had signed the order upon my request. At first he was reluctant to do this, and as a result she was suffering needlessly. The liquid would get into her lungs little by little. This was confirmed by the nurse who told me that the lower part of her lungs did not work. It was my interpretation that the forced feedings had created this problem. I had witnesses who told me that the nursing staff forced her to take food. I also found bibs if they were left on her bedcover. They were usually moist and covered with spots. I would also see spots on her sheets where she would spit the liquids out. Patients who had the full capacity of their brains were not treated like this. They pushed the food off the tray, hit the spoon, or used their hands to prevent feeding, or spit the food at the staff. My wife would not do this. Relatives who do not visit that often tell the staff, "Pinch her nose; she has to eat or take medication."

Suddenly there was a knock on the door and I left these sad memories behind. The hospice volunteer had arrived. This volunteer would stay and sit with Christina if I was unavailable. I had met Carol at the nursing home, where the staffing during the three-to-eleven shift was bad, very bad. Agency Aides and LPNs were hired, but the chronic shortage was evident every day. Being there and watching what went on, I knew my wife would be a victim of these personnel policies. I had asked the hospice center at the nursing home to get a volunteer to be with my wife when I could not be there to ensure that she got the care she needed.

I had met Carol in the hall of the nursing home just before my morning visit with my wife. She stepped forward and greeted me. We had gone to my wife's room, where I told her more about what was going on the nursing home. The shortage was not only in this nursing home, but all across the country. Carol was not a stranger to this. She knew because her mother had died at the nursing home. She had also lost her father and husband. She would visit after I left in the evening to see that my wife would not be forgotten. If you cannot talk and complain, who will speak up for you? Carol watched over my wife, even after all she had gone through herself. What a great lady. Carol told me she was quite impressed with the hospice center. She had heard a lot of good things about it.

If you have seen nursing homes and then you come to a hospice center you see the vast difference between the two. Nursing homes are built like hospitals. This is not right. The difference in use is too great. Maybe some architect will wake up and build a nursing home that will meet the needs of this rapidly growing but forgotten and neglected portion of the population.

The hospice building was not large, but it gave the feeling of space and light. There were no narrow halls with rooms on the left and right side. It had a kitchen where relatives could cook a meal and eat it as conveniently as at home. It was tastefully decorated. The furniture was of excellent quality. One large room had a fireplace. Some of the windows had beautiful stained glass like you see in churches. There was wall-to-wall carpeting in the private rooms and throughout the whole building, with designs in it to break the monotony. My wife's room was wonderful, too, as I described earlier. Carol said this place felt like a home. Yes, I responded, but an expensive one. Before she sat down, she asked me if I wanted a cup of coffee. When she returned with the coffee cups, she took a chair and sat down on the other side of the bed. I explained to Carol what had happened to get Christina to the hospice center. We talked for some time when she suddenly realized she had to go to pick up a friend. I expressed my appreciation for all that she had done for my wife. It was quiet in the room again.

I looked at my wife; she had a different look. Her eyes were still closed and her lips were open, but there was something different. I did not know what it was, or maybe it was just me? The nurse came in and gave Christina her daily bath. I stayed in the room as I had done in the nursing home. There should have been two aides in the nursing home according to her care plan, but there never were. I was always the number two. When they turned my wife on her side, I noticed that the open sore had become larger and around this sore was a red ring of skin. It did look very bad—a large wound without skin, tissue slowly disappearing and leaving an empty space. The tissue was dissolving into body fluid, which had a terrible odor. I looked at her face—no change—but then I noticed the edge of her right ear was red. It was red from lying too long on that side, so I asked the nurses to look at it. They made a ring of cotton with surgical tape to fit under her ear. They also put Vaseline on the ear and elevated her head so the ear would not touch the pillow. In the afternoon, I looked at her face, and it had changed. She had a different expression on her face, and I did not know why. Her hands were cold, so I warmed them. I checked her feet, and they were cold as well. I left to get a cup of coffee, and when I got back, her hands were cold again. I placed another blanket on her. When the evening shift came on duty, the nurse commented, "I can see the change."

This proved to me that my observation had been right.

It was a hopeless feeling, that I could do so little to make the end of her life more comfortable. I could still put Vaseline on her lips and try to warm her hands, but they would get cold as soon as I left. Another blanket would not help. I was very sad and depressed. My remaining comfort would be to keep holding her hands and being with her. I knew she felt my presence. She knew I was there and stayed as long as I could.

I left that afternoon very, very unhappy and depressed and lost. The next morning I came in and checked her. I saw that she had medical tape on her upper arm and two small plastic tubes sticking out. They were ports, one for drawing blood and one for pain medication. I put Vaseline on her lips and the edge of her ear.

I adjusted the cotton ring around her ear. I went to the kitchen to get water and coffee.

Christina's hands were cold but her feet were warm, so I was happy about that. There was no change in her face. She had the same strange expression—lips open, eyes closed.

Many nurses, social workers and counselors, and a female chaplain had visited us, but no doctor. So when Christina's hands were warm, I went to the office and asked to see the doctor. The doctor was busy, but I was told she would meet me in my wife's room. The doctor and a supervisor came to the room and examined Christina. The doctor commented, "She has a strong heart." This was no surprise to me. I heard that comment after every examination. The doctor began talking about Christina's illness and current condition. It took some time before I had a chance to speak. "Doctor, this is not what I want to talk about. It is about what to put on her death certificate." I was quite sure that this came as a surprise to her. Christina's regular doctor was on vacation; this one was just filling in. This doctor had just told me that my wife had a strong heart; yet, if Christina were to die before her regular doctor returned, this doctor would put heart failure as the cause of death on Christina's death certificate. This doctor, like most doctors, did not want to put on the death certificate, when the time came, that the disease of Alzheimer's killed my wife. We talked a little about my wife, and then they left.

The nurses were late this morning. I looked at the open sore; the smell was really bad. One nurse said, "The pharmacist will provide some powder for the odor." They also had two syringes of morphine that were administered directly into the port. One nurse commented, "It is good to see this that you love her so much."

The attending doctor told me the name of the doctor in charge this weekend. There would be two nurses for the bathing. The counselors, social workers, and administrative personnel did not work on the weekends. In other words, it would be a skeleton crew, just as in the nursing home. The supervisor could call for assistance if needed. When I was ready to leave, I brought my coffee cup and glass to the kitchen and met two nurses there. I told them that

Monday would be a bad traffic day. The overpass was going to close so they could lay concrete beams over the support columns. The trucks and cranes would be on the highway under the overpass and blocking the whole intersection for five days. I asked how I could get around that. They suggested I take a road that runs parallel to the highway. I should go through a development, make a right at the second traffic light, and then a left and I would be on the road that runs parallel with the highway. I thanked them and said I would make a dry run on Saturday.

Saturday morning, I tried the new route and it was simple, just as the nurse had said. It was an unjustified fear I had, not knowing exactly how the newly constructed highway with the new under—and overpasses would work. Should I get off at this intersection or the next? I was an expert at making the wrong turns. If I had to go right I always took a left turn and vice versa. I was happy this unjustified fear was gone.

The early Saturday traffic is very light. I told myself from then on I would avoid the construction on the overpass and use the new highway to get to the hospice. Another surprise was the parking lot on the weekend. During the week, I could not find a place to park and had to park outside the parking area on a dead-end road. Now I could park close to the door. The door was locked, so I rang the doorbell and looked through the window. There was no receptionist at the desk, but a voice answered. I said I was here to visit my wife; I got no response but heard a "buzzing" noise. I tried to open the door but it was locked. I flagged someone down inside who was walking through the hall.

I bought breakfast for the staff, but I did not see anyone. I went to Christina's room and checked on her. The pillow between her knees was missing. Her right leg had been contracted for some time as a result of malnutrition. The nursing home had placed a regular bed pillow between her knees, but this usually slipped out. I designed one for my wife. I purchased an egg-crate pillow and cut six inches off. I put a plastic grocery bag on one end and the overlap was rolled around and taped so that there would not be any wrinkles. Then I did the other side, overlapping the first bag, and taped the two bags together so that no fluid could wet the inside. A pillow case overlapping and without wrinkles was put over the egg-crate pillow and put between her knees to prevent pressure sores. I looked around. The only place the pillow could be was in her linen cabinet. so I opened the door and there it was. I put it in between her knees and checked her feet, which were cold. I put Vaseline on her lips and ear. As usual, her eyes were closed and her mouth was open. There was nothing I could do about her feet. Christina had as many covers as possible. I took her hands and held them, and stroked her hands and cheeks. Touching is very important. When speech is not possible anymore, physical contact can be the only communication. I did not keep track of time, but I noticed a slight warming of her hands, so I changed the order in which I held her hands. I kept one hand on her body and stroked the free hand. So far, this system had always worked, and it worked this time too.

I went to the kitchen to get coffee and water, because I could smell the coffee brewing. Back in her room I adjusted the cotton ring around her ear. I noticed that her breathing was different. This was not the first time. I watched it slowing down till I could hardly notice her chest going up or down. It did not last long, and then it seemed to make up for the slowdown with rapid movements. Then it was back to normal. Her hands were still warm, so I put a CD on and drank the coffee and watched her as I had done for so many years.

I did not know what time it was when the nurses arrived to give Christina her bath. When they rolled her over to do her back, I noticed that the open sore was larger. The tissue was disappearing, dissolving, draining, and that part of her body was gone forever, leaving an open, empty space never to be replaced. She got her two injections of morphine. She still had her eyes closed and her mouth open. The nurses checked her cotton ear ring, which I had just taken care of.

When I returned in the afternoon, it was the usual scene I saw every day, except there were no staff members coming in to visit. I did the same thing—watched Christina, kept her hands warm, listened to the music, drank coffee and water, stroked her cheeks, and talked to her.

Today was a week from the day that I had gone to the nursing home to prevent them from force-feeding her, so Christina had gone for an entire week with no food or drink. Ever since Christina went into the nursing home, I had always given her dinner. It saved the staff time, but no one ever expressed appreciation for this free service. She had a good appetite, but never ate large portions. When the dinner tray came, I would taste the food and if I did not like it, I did not feed that particular part of the evening dinner to her. In addition, I brought in baby food jars to replace the items she did not like. I was never in a hurry to feed her. The nursing-home style is quite different, and some of the patients who do not like what is offered take this out on the aides. As always, there are caring nurses' aides who do take the time to feed the patients properly.

When there is a shortage of staff, everyone suffers, but the ones who cannot speak for themselves are at the tail end of the line for help. On the other side, there are the ones who eat and succeed in getting more food. This group can be easily identified by looking at their stomachs.

We had living wills at the time we moved to Pennsylvania, but they had to be modified to the laws of the state. My wife and I discussed in the past that if we were hurt or injured or had an incurable illness, we did not want to live longer through artificial means. We also had a DNR (Do Not Resuscitate) order and we both had the authority to make medical decisions for each other. During the seven nursing-home years, I had made the decision for Christina that as long as she accepted food from me, I would give it to her, but if she refused to accept food or fluid from me, I would consider this a sign that she did not want to live anymore. During my observations in those years, I have seen that this is, most of the time, denied or ignored by the nursing staff.

Patients in severe pain feel when the time to die is approaching, and all they want is to ease the pain. Most doctors do not have training in pain management, or palliative or hospice care. This is a crying shame. I had heard that you could live more than seven days without food or water.

I was home for only a short while that day when the doorbell rang. In our neighborhood, people do not call on others when it is dark. Most of the neighbors are retired and were raised on farms, so they still go to bed early. Around 10 p.m., most lights are turned off in these homes. So I was surprised when I saw our daughter Ellen. She usually works on Saturdays and had driven many hours to get here. We kissed each other and I said, "I was going to prepare a sandwich, but now let's go out to eat. I hardly ever do that, so let's live it up."

We drove to the nearest restaurant, but that one was very crowded and had a long line for seating. We decided to go to another restaurant. Some people looked at us when we walked out. The other restaurant was about four miles out of town and we got seated right away. I told my daughter in more detail about her mother and what had happened in the nursing home the week before and how angry and upset I was. The food at this place was always good, not fancy, and the service was pleasant. We talked more and also when we got home. Before we knew it, it was quite late, and I told my daughter, "I have to be at the hospice early, but you sleep as long as you want and meet me at the hospice," and I told her how to get there.

The Sunday morning ride to the hospice was pleasant. The sun was out, and the temperature was in the forties. It was very mild for January. It was the second day that I could park next to the building entrance. Two people came out the door to light up their cigarettes, so I did not have to use the doorbell. I walked through the long wide hall. Nobody was visible when I passed the kitchen, but I could smell the coffee.

I did my routine checking, and when I kissed her forehead, it was cold. Her eyes were closed, her mouth was open, and her lips were dry. No reaction, the same. I put Vaseline on her lips and her ear, rearranged her cotton ring, turned the pillow, and checked her ear again. Her feet were warm. I went to the kitchen to get coffee and water. I returned with my coffee, selected a CD, and took my wife's hands to warm them in the usual way.

The nurses came in early and washed Christina. They turned her on her side and the red ring on the outside of the wound looked different. Where the skin had completely disappeared, you could see tissue and empty spaces and the smell was bad. I knew it would get worse and worse every day she lived; however, the terrible pain caused by this process was partially compensated for by the morphine.

The hospice nurses are given time to provide excellent care for the patients. It is not like in the nursing-home industry, where all patient activities are scheduled with limited time frames.

In spite of these sad memories of the past which will not go away, in this place I felt at ease. I knew that Christina's pain medication was working for her and the nursing staff was very responsive to her needs. While these memories were running through my head, our daughter Ellen came in the room and saw her mother in a condition she had never seen her before. It made her very sad. I am sure she knew that her mother was dying and this was the last time she would see her alive. We watched her silently.

Then suddenly the phone rang. It was our son Olof who had arrived and was calling from our home to get directions on how to reach the hospice. I told him about the new way I used and mentioned that since it was past noon, we would go out to their favorite restaurant and after lunch return to the hospice. It would be at least thirty minutes before my son arrived, so I said to my daughter, "I will leave you alone with your mother." and left the room.

I took a more detailed look at the building—the conference rooms, the meeting rooms, the library, and the kitchen with its latest electrical range, the cabinets with dishes, glasses, and everything you need to serve a meal. I poured myself another cup of coffee and sat down in the room with the fireplace so I could see our son coming.

When he arrived, we greeted each other, and he was surprised to see how beautiful this hospice was. We have a fireplace at home, but not in such a spacious room as this. I showed him where the kitchen was so he could make himself a cup of tea. He knew that his sister was already in the room, and when he entered he was startled to see his mother's condition. He did visit his mother at regular intervals, so this sight was a great shock to him. I sat on the sofa and our children sat on the two chairs that were in the room. There was no change; her eyes were closed and her mouth was open. Our daughter was keeping her mother's hands warm, and I put Vaseline on her lips and right ear.

Our son and daughter had had no breakfast, so they were eager to get some food. There was an Indian restaurant close by. Our son had found this restaurant when he came for visits to the nursing home. In the beginning, we ordered from the menu, but we soon found out that it took close to an hour to get a special dish and eat it. This was too much time for me to be away from the nursing home. From that time on, we used only the buffet, which had a large variety of tasty dishes. You also could go back for seconds.

We returned to the hospice after lunch and I checked Christina's hands. They were not cold, but sweaty hot. I got a wash cloth out of her linen cabinet and soaked it with cold water. I placed this on her forehead. This seemed to bring down her temperature a bit.

Our daughter told us that there was a good opportunity for her to get a position at a small corporate international airport. The corporate jets flew from all parts of the world, returning from meetings at their production facilities. My daughter also had three small children, our grandchildren, ages eleven, eight and six. They were home now with her husband, but she needed to get back to her family. I asked our son if he wanted to stay with his mother a while longer. My daughter would follow me through the labyrinths of detours in the construction zone of the highways, which had gone on now for three years. I reapplied Christina's cold compress; she was cooling down now. Our daughter and I left and our son would stay with his mother.

The next morning when I arrived at the hospice building, the parking lot was empty again. I knew that yesterday was Sunday, so it must be a holiday. Holidays did not mean much to me anymore. In all those years at the nursing home, it just meant less than the usual understaffed help. Here at the hospice there were always enough nurses to take care of the patients. I checked my wife's condition. Her forehead and face were cold; her hands were warm. I put Vaseline on her lips and the edge of her ear.

The nurses came in early today with their linen cart and washed her. When they turned her on her side, I saw the open sore. It looked terrible. The red ring around the open sore was now larger and more tissue inside was gone. There was emptiness and the odor was bad. The gauze pads used before had to be replaced by larger ones. The sore continued to get larger and larger. It looked like a crater. The doctor had told me that every day the tissue would dissolve and drain away. It was like the saying, "Life is draining away." This was now true for my wife. Slowly the tissue would disappear; there was no stopping this process and the pain and discomfort would be terrible. Christina got a lot of morphine to keep her sedated. Her body did not receive nutrition anymore so it started to use what was available. Fat and muscle were being consumed to keep the body alive. After observing this, I went to the sitting area, took a chair, and sat down. I watched the nurses finishing her daily bath and treatment, including the morphine containers to control the pain. After the nurses had left, I moved the chair close to her bed and held her hands and stroked her cheeks. I knew she could feel my presence, and I talked to her as I had done for all these years.

One of the other nurses came in and told me that no one on staff had expected my wife to make it through the weekend, but she did. This reminded me of another event that occurred many years ago. I got a call from the nursing home asking me to come over because the staff did not expect her to make it. I still remember the drive to the nursing home, telling myself this was the last time I would see her alive. Emotions bubbled up and tears came to my eyes, so I slowed down a bit to keep control of the car. When I got to her room that day, there were a lot of medical personnel standing around her bed. I did the same thing. I took her hands and talked to her. She did not pass, though. She lived for quite a few years.

In the afternoon, the attending doctor arrived. She was a pleasant woman. She mentioned first that the drainage of the sore had increased over the weekend. She told me about her family and that she had just returned from a short vacation with her family in the mountains. I told her about our family and my wife's illness, which started to show after we moved, after she was exposed to a new environment. Alzheimer's cannot be prevented by keeping your body and mind active in your youth. Alzheimer's knows no social, sexual, ethnic, or educational boundaries. Alzheimer's is also the most over diagnosed illness. Twenty-five percent who carry this label do not have it. Then I stopped, because I knew the doctor was a specialist in geriatrics.

"Doctor, I read that on death certificates, where it asks for the immediate cause, final disease, or condition resulting in death, Alzheimer's is hardly ever recorded. Yet we have over diagnosed 25 percent of the cases. This is a discrepancy, and let me explain why I want to have this illness recorded for her. Christina's parent, grandparents, and great-grandparents all died in their sleep and were in their eighties and nineties. In our country in the beginning of the 1900s, the average life expectancy was fifty years. She was never ill. The only times she was in the hospital was to deliver our children, and that time she enjoyed, which was about a week. All that has happened to her in the nursing home was a result of her illness and could have been treated differently if the quality of care had been much better. Her heart, lungs, digestive, and urinary systems have been in good shape. My wife's only problem was that her brain was slowly dying as a result of Alzheimer's. Would you please record this on her death certificate?" She did not answer, but I knew she would do it.

On Tuesday, the parking lot was full, so I had to park on the dead-end street. When I came to Christina's room, there was, as usual, no change. Her face, her forehead, and her hands were warm. I put Vaseline on her lips and her ear. She did not move. It did not take long before the nurses came in to wash her. When they came, I always moved my chair to a spot from which I could see her back with the open sore. This morning, I could not believe what I saw. Tissue under the red, round perimeter of the wound was gone, yes gone. There was no skin attached to the underlying tissue; it was hanging loose all around the edges. When the nurses pulled her gently over, the skin moved with the turning of her body. It was a terrifying sight. The open wound had been infected for some time. It had started in the nursing home, and it smelled bad. The emptiness, tissue dissolving slowly, draining away, like her life draining away. Her face showed the terrible pain and discomfort, and the nurses saw it, too. Christina did not utter a sound. Her facial expression did all the talking. I walked over to her side and took her hand and stroked her forehead and cheeks. The nurses went to her medicine cabinet and filled the two containers with morphine. That was all they could do, and I did my part by comforting her as best as I could. The nurses were silent as they walked out of the room. The hospice staff had inherited this open-sore problem. They did what they could, but it was too late.

I was so mentally exhausted that I had to lie down on the sofa, but in such a way that I could still see Christina's face. She did not move. Suddenly I heard a very big sigh from her and jumped up, but she was quiet again. I sat down next to her and watched her, but I saw no movement. I checked her respiration, but it was normal. Her eyes were closed and her lips were open, so I waited for quite some time, and then I went back to the sofa, still keeping an eye on her. I must have slept for a while, because when I woke up it was time for me to go home.

The next morning, driving to the hospice, I was suddenly overwhelmed with a great feeling. I don't know what this was about, but without these bursts of good feeling, I never could have survived all these years in the condition I am in now. It made me sing if I had the radio on and knew the words of the song. All troubles seemed to flow away—no anger about our lousy health-care system, but contentment, a personal happiness. First it would peak and fade a bit, but then it would stay with me. It gave me a lift for a short time, a much needed one. It is like while you are flying above the clouds, nothing but the blue sky and the white puffy clouds below you. Then I would ask myself, *How can you feel this way when your wife is dying? She might not make it that long. Why should you be happy?* But that thinking lasted for only a sort while. It was a great feeling, and it stayed. It was like a curve; it reached a high point, and then it went slowly down during the day. It was in this spirit that I entered the hospice this morning.

When I came into Christina's room and looked at her, there were tears in her eyes. I had not seen this in quite some time, so I took a tissue and dried her eyes. There was a very short reaction while I did this. I checked the Vaseline; there was just enough left for this morning. There was no reaction when I put the Vaseline on her lips and ear. Her hands were warm. When a nurse came in, I showed her the empty tube. I asked her if she could get some more; it was called scope gel. She returned with the gel and another nurse to wash Christina. I went to the kitchen to get coffee and water. After the nurses had done their job, one of the counselors came in. We had met before in the first days, and I told her about my wife's condition and that it was getting worse. She knew all about it. When I was still talking and looking at my wife, I turned my eyes to her and saw tears in her eyes. She was a counselor and also a sensitive, caring person who let her emotions go freely and did not keep up the professional dignity. I liked that very much in her.

When I returned in the afternoon, Christina's hands were warm and sweaty, but her feet and knees were cold. Her thighs were warm. Her hands were slack, no grip at all. Later, the two nurses came in and rolled her over gently to measure the size of the open sore, which became larger every day. More skin and underlying tissue was disappearing. Shortly after that, the doctor came in to check my wife's pulse, and she told me she could hardly hear it and left. I sat next to my wife, lost, my mind blank. When you are in a condition like this, you have lost your objectivity. Fear and sorrow take over, and the good feeling of the morning was gone.

It was after nine o'clock in the evening when I got a call from the hospice. "There is a change; please come," I was told When I got to Christina's room, there was a nurse sitting by the bed who reported that her breathing had become irregular. The hospice/nursing-home volunteer soon showed up, and she sat with me. I expressed my appreciation, and we watched Christina together. I was holding my wife's hands under the blankets to keep them warm. Her respiration was irregular, but after some time it became regular again. It reminded me of the many times Christina had had a close call in the nursing home and the staff did not expect her to live but she did. I shared this with the volunteer. When it was well past midnight I told the volunteer that I felt my wife was stable and I would go home. She said she would stay another few hours just to make sure there was no change. I expressed my gratitude and left.

Early the next morning, as I was getting ready to leave for the hospice, the phone rang. Christina had just died. They asked me if I wanted to see her. I said, "Of course." I came in the room and looked at her. Her eyes were closed and her lips were open, but now her whole body was absolutely still and cold. I kissed her for the last time and stayed with her for quite some time.

All her suffering and pain were gone.

AFTERWORD

Ellen van Amstel-Oates

First and foremost, I want to thank my father for taking the time to write this account of my mother's illness. Christina's disease devastated our family. It was absolute heartbreak, especially for the man who loved her so unconditionally.

The love and devotion my parents bestowed upon each other and our family is the greatest gift I have received in my life. I am proud and grateful to be the daughter of Gerard and Christina van Amstel.

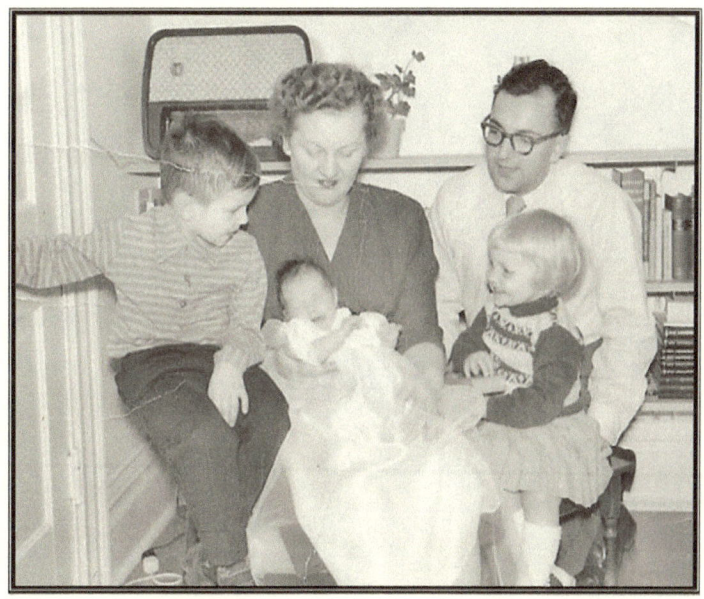

Christina, Gerard, Olof, Karen, and Ellen